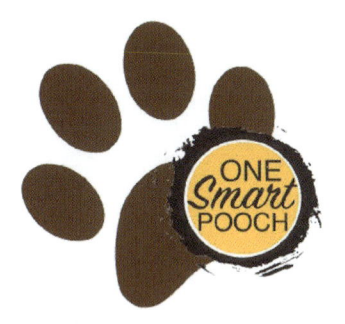

Pet CPR & First Aid Care

For Canine and Felines

Note: This information is *not* meant to be a substitute for care by a veterinarian!
If you have any concerns or questions about your pet's health, please see your veterinarian, immediately!
Most Veterinarians cannot bring your pet back to life, but by knowing First-Aid & CPR, you can keep your pet alive until you reach a Veterinarian.

By knowing Pet First-Aid you can/could:

- Lower your pet's body temperature if your pet is suffering from Heat Stroke, preventing brain damage or death.
- Artificially keep your pet's heart and lungs working until you can get your pet to a veterinarian.
- Prevent your pet from losing consciousness by alleviating choking.
- Expel poisons from your pet's system by properly inducing vomiting.
- Stop bleeding from an open wound or cut.
- Prevent infection by knowing how to properly bandaging and cleaning a wound.

By learning what can or could happen to your pet, you can prevent most emergencies!

First-aid is NOT a substitute for professional veterinary care!
You and your Veterinarian must work together as a team for the health of your pet and to keep your pet healthy!

Pet First-Aid & Human First-Aid

Pet First-Aid is the first step in an attempt to make your pet more comfortable. Providing the proper comfort will lower the risk of infection and could even stop further injuries!

Canine and feline anatomy is *not* the same as ours.

A big difference between human and animal first aid and CPR is animals bite!

The differences between treating humans and your pet:

Our pets can't tell us where they hurt.

Our pets can't tell us why they hurt.

Our pets anatomy/physiology is different from ours.

Examples: When performing rescue breathing on a human, you could pinch the nose shut and breathe into the person's mouth. With your pet, you would do the opposite, close your pet's mouth and breathe into the nostrils to obtain the best flow into the airway.

Animals do not speak English and since we can't ask our pets, "What's wrong or hurting?", plus they often hide signs of injury or illness from the other pack members we, as the pet owner, have to play detective to find out what's wrong on with our pet.

Notes: Learning how to appropriately restrain and handle an injured or sick pet is very important, also. You will learn more how to appropriately restrain and handle your sick or injured pet. If you get injured, there will be nothing you can do for your injured pet.

Animals that are known to have bitten someone or another animal should be quarantine until seen by a licensed veterinarian!

Facts: Sometimes without warning tragedy can strike and knowing what to do could save your pets life! Statistics show that preventable accidents are a leading cause of deaths among our pets and 9 out of 10 pets can expect to have an emergency during their lifetime. According to the American Animal Hospital Association (AAHA), 1 out of 4 pets could have been saved if just one Pet First-Aid technique was applied prior to seeing a veterinarian.

Assessing an Emergency Situation

Assessing an emergency situation is known as *Triage*.

Triage is the process of evaluating the needs of an animal during an emergency.

Note: When there's more than one animal to evaluate the order of importance for providing assistance is to the most critically in need animal.

Meaning, the animals in life threatening conditions get seen/treated first!

No matter if it's your pet or an human friend, you should always ask yourself these 3 questions in this order when evaluating an emergency situation:

1. Is the animal breathing? Heart is working, but the lungs have stopped functioning. The absence of breathing is considered a life-threatening emergency! Always check for breathing first.

Note: You need to perform Rescue Breathing right away!

If your pet is breathing, skip to question 3. If your pet's breathing the heart is beating.

2. Has the heart stopped beating? No pulse can be detected and the animal has stopped breathing. When an animal's heart stops beating within a matter of minutes, irreparable cell damage can occur.

Note: This is **always** considered a life-threatening emergency! You must begin CPR -- Cardio Pulmonary Resuscitation right away! You will learn more later on in the book.

3. Is the animal in any physical distress? Heart & lungs are working but something is still wrong. Distress may range from mild digestive upset to unconsciousness, choking, bleeding, seizures, burns, and more.

Note: Physical distress, depending on the type can be life-threatening!

The type of distress will determine the type of first-aid to administer.

11 Situations that will Always Require seeing your Veterinarian

No matter what first-aid technique you decide to perform to make your pet more comfortable, for the injuries listed below you must see your veterinarian immediately!

"If in doubt, please get advice from your licensed veterinarian!"

1. Trauma to head and/or face, chest and/or abdomen, or anytime an animal has been unconscious at any period or time.

2. First-time Seizure, a seizure that last more than five minutes.

Note: In cases of an epileptic animal, a seizure lasting longer than normal!

3. Arterial bleeding or bright red spurting bleeding.

4. Suspected muscle/tendon strains/tears and/or fractures.

5. Wounds that are more than 1" in length and/or ½" deep including bites, cuts, and puncture wounds.

6. Suspected snake bites.

7. Suspect a condition known as Shock.

Note: You will learn more about shock later on in the book.
8. Anytime you have to administer Rescue Breathing and/or CPR or any signs of Respiratory distress.
9. Inability to walk.
10. Suspect a condition known as Bloat.
   Note: You will learn more about bloat later on it the book.
11. Suspected of poisoning.

Assessing your Pet's Health
Learning to check your pet's vitals can help assess their level of pain, injury or illness!
Here's how you check your pet's vitals:
1. Pulse – The rhythmic movement of blood through an artery.
• Place the ball of two fingers, pointer and middle finger, on the depression found on the upper inner thigh over your pet's Femoral Artery.
• Count the beats for 6 seconds and then add a zero to the end of how many beats counted. Count the beats for 30 seconds and then multiply by 2. Count the beats for 60 seconds to determine your pet's pulse rate. If you have difficulty feeling the Femoral Artery, place the palm of your hand over the left side of your pet's chest just behind the elbow to feel for a heartbeat.

ONE SMART POOCH

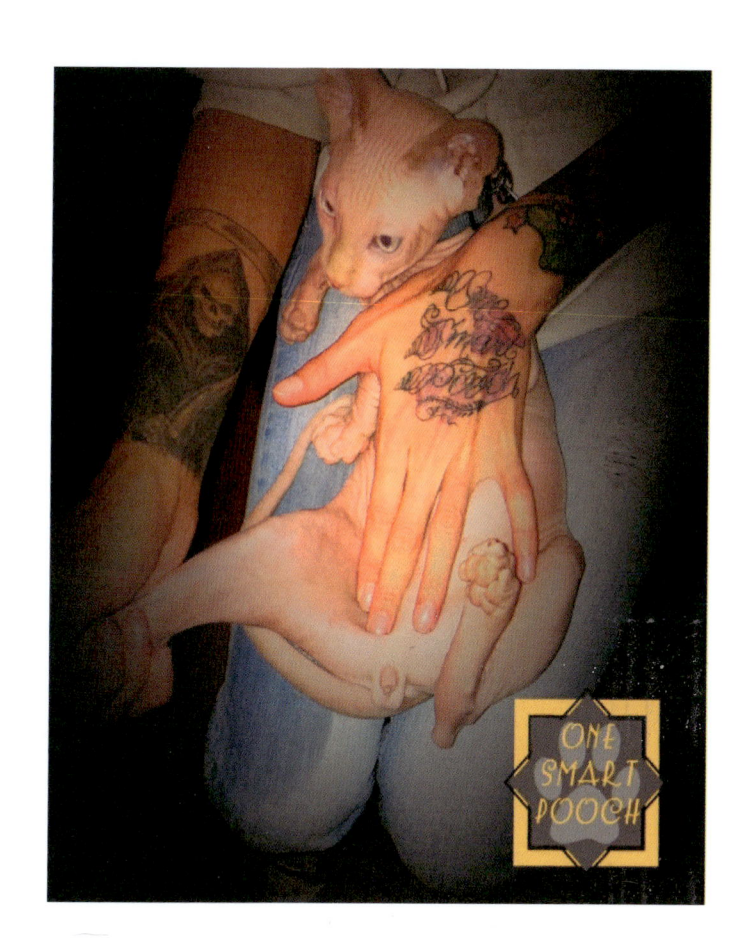

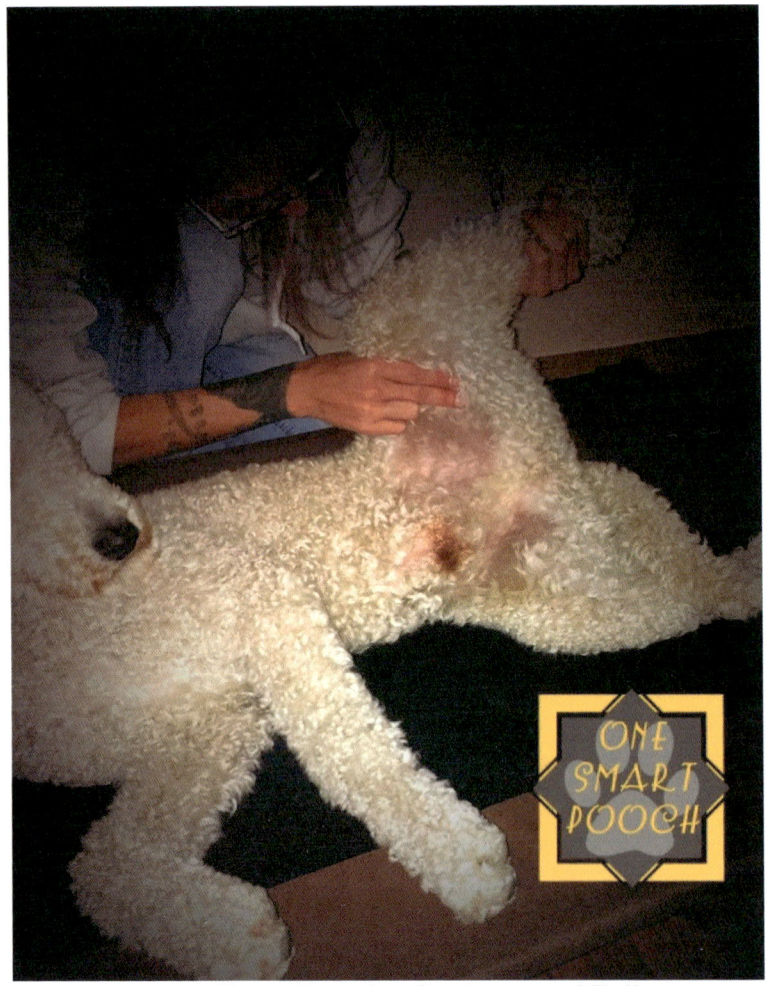

Average Heart Rate for Canines and Felines
Felines, 160 – 200 beats per minute
Small Canines, 90 – 160 beats per minute
Medium to Large canines, 65 – 90 beats per minute

2. Respiration – The process of inhaling and exhaling; breathing.

• Place your hand over your pet's chest to count the number of times his/her chest rises or falls. A rises is an inhale and a fall is an exhale. The "rise and fall cycle" should be counted as one breath.

• Count the breaths for 60 seconds or for 30 seconds and then multiply by 2 to determine your pet's respirations per minute.

Note: Do *NOT* count the respirations of a panting canine or feline if you do your respirations per minute will be incorrect.

Very large canines and/or geriatric animals may have slower respirations.

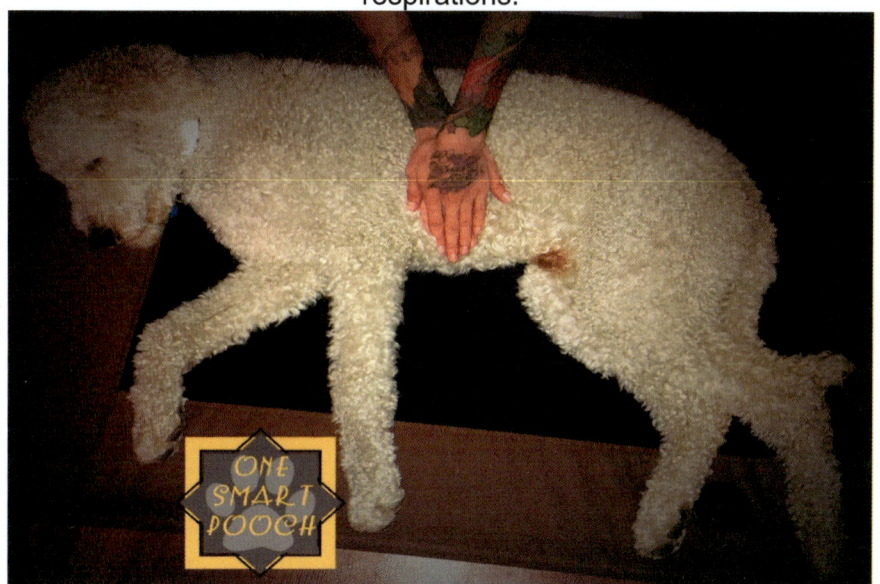

Average Respiration Rate for Dogs and Cats
Felines and Small Canines, 20 – 40 breaths per minute
Medium to Large Canines, 10 – 30 breaths per minute

3. Temperature – The level of heat produced by the body.
• After lubricating the tip of a digital thermometer with petroleum jelly, lift your pet's tail up and insert thermometer 1 into the rectum, slightly angled upward toward his/her spin.
• At the sound of the beep or according to specific instrument instructions given within the package of the thermometer read your pet's temperature.
   Note: The average animal's temperature range should between 100.0 F – 102.5 F and 38 C – 39.16 C.
• The temperature of 103 F is considered a fever.
• The temperature of 104 F and above is considered an emergency.
   Note: Feeling your pet's nose to determine his/her temperature is *not* accurate!

4. CRT or Capillary Refill Time – The amount of time it takes for blood and oxygen to refill a capillary. CRT indicates whether blood circulation is sufficient to sustain life.
• Gently lift your pet's upper lip then press on gums above teeth using the ball of your index finger until gums lighten.

Note: Be sure *NOT* to pull too tight on your pet's lip because this can cause the gums to appear lighter making it more difficult to accurately assess the CRT.

• It's best to choose a non-pigmented or the lights part of your pet's gums, if possible.

Note: If you only have dark gums to work with, you should still be able to determine your pet's CRT.

• Release the pressure on the gums and the color should return to normal within 1-2 seconds.

Note: If it takes the color longer than 2 to 5 seconds to return to normal, increase circulation by slightly elevating your pet's hind quarters with a pillow and immediate get to your veterinarian for help.

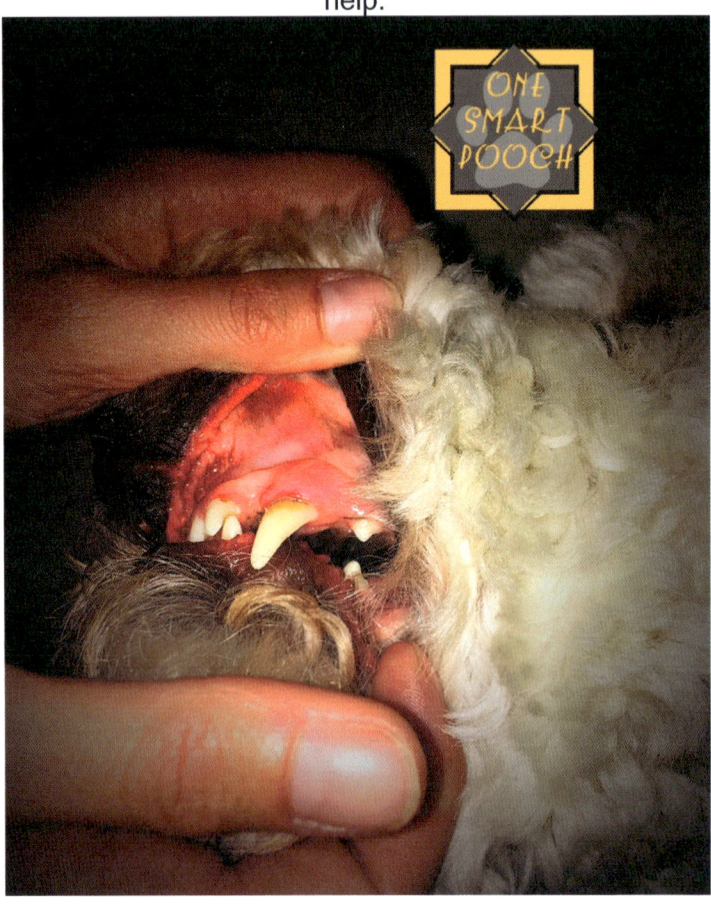

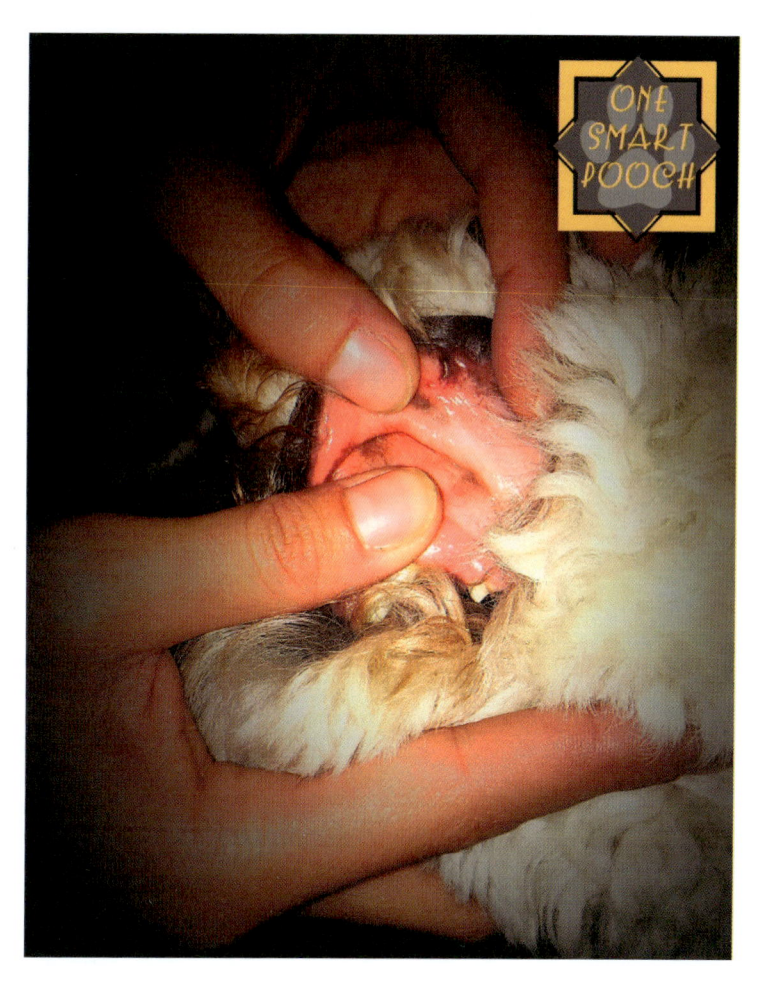

Note: *Do NOT elevate your pet's hind quarters if there's significant bleeding to the head or chest!*

5. Hydration – Sufficient water in an animal's body to sustain life. Dehydration is the loss of water and vital electrolytes like sodium, chloride and potassium that an animal needs for survival.

Facts: Canines and felines are comprised of 70% to 80% water. Canines and felines are very resilient and can survive up to 50% of their muscle/fat loss.

To determine adequate hydration levels, follow the following steps:
• Gently pinch a fold of the skin at your pet's nape of their neck and release.

Notes: The skin should quickly fall back into place, your pet is hydrated.

- For loose-skinned breeds like a Shar Pei and/or older pets, that's skin may have lost elasticity, carefully feel the animal's gums.

Notes: If the gums are dry and/or sticky, your pet may be dehydrated.

Fatigue, constipation, increased heart rate and sunken eyes can also be a sign of dehydration.

Fact: A dehydration level of more than 10% is life threatening for a canine or feline.

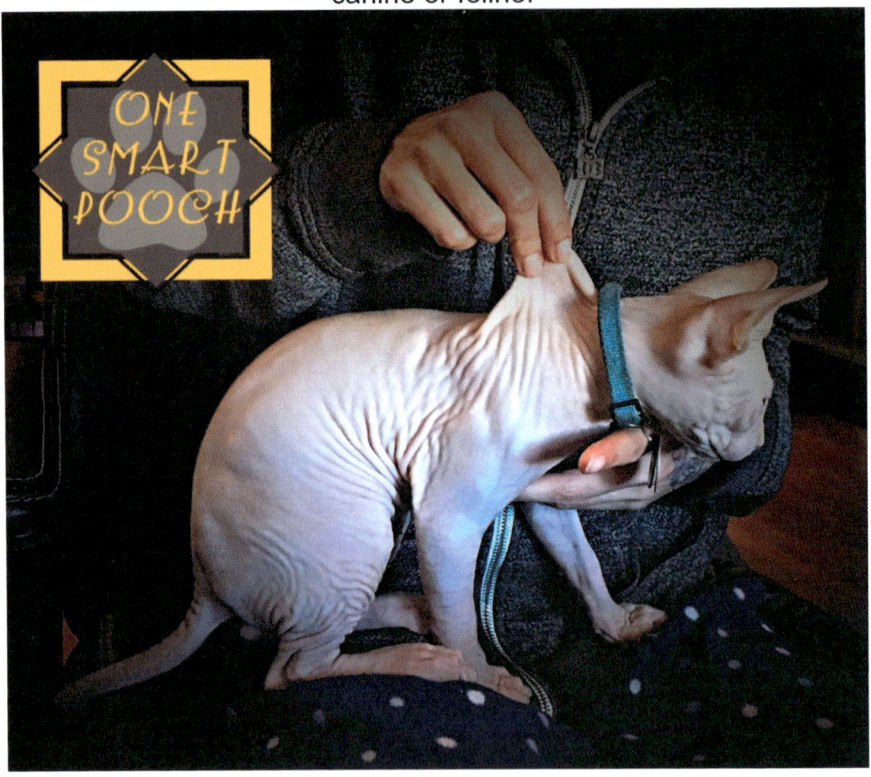

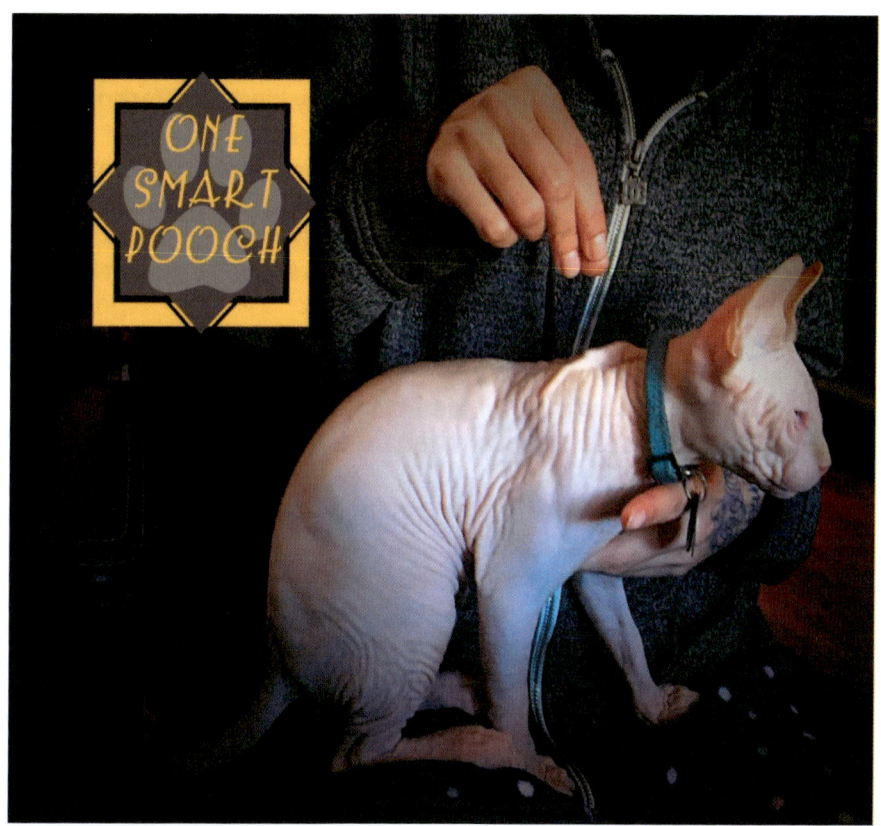

Examining from Head-to-Tail

After checking your pet's vitals, it's important to observe the animal's body for any signs of injuries or illnesses. The key to recognizing something that is not right or wrong with your pet is to know what's normal for any feline or canine.

We suggest starting at the head and work your way toward the tail. Observe the skin and coat, feeling for any lumps, bumps, abrasions and/or parasites. Look for any redness or tender areas on your pet's body. Watch for how your pet reacts to your touch as you do your examination.

Note: Canines are more tolerant to a painful touch. Felines will immediately let you know that is bothering them, if your touch hurts.

~Gently clean your pet's *ears* of dirt and/or wax with ear wash or a soft wash cloth.
If you see redness, parasites or smell a foul odor call your Veterinarian.

Before you perform first-aid, you may have to muzzle the animal or wrap him/her up in a towel to safely offer assistance. Even the sweetest of animals may bite when he/she is scared, stressed, or in pain.

Note: Animals are very perceptive on picking up on our emotions and if you do not feel confident enough to help, you are better off getting your pet to someone who can help!

Restraining Techniques
Most importantly, you need to be in control!
~Chase your pet into a room or enclosed area.

Note: You may have to move some furniture before you can get to your pet.

~Small pets may settle down best if you wrap them in a towel.

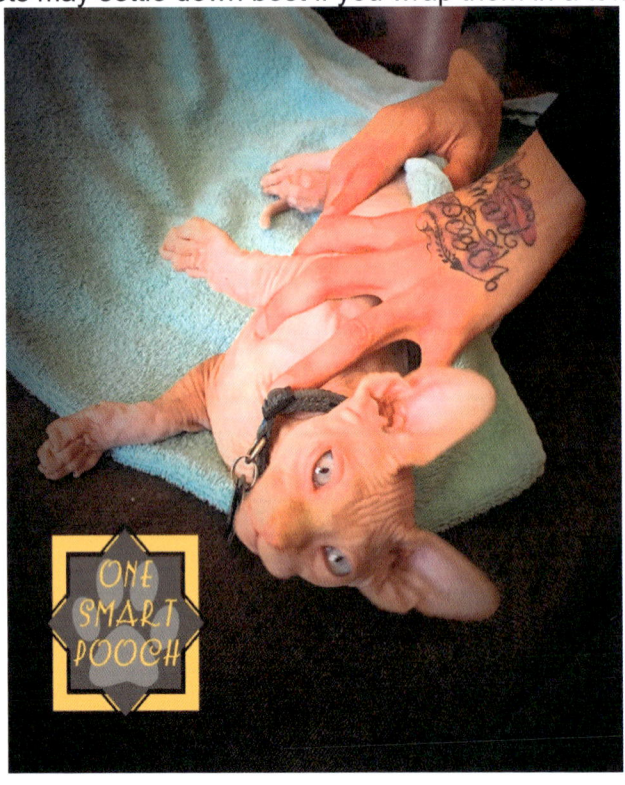

ONE SMART POOCH

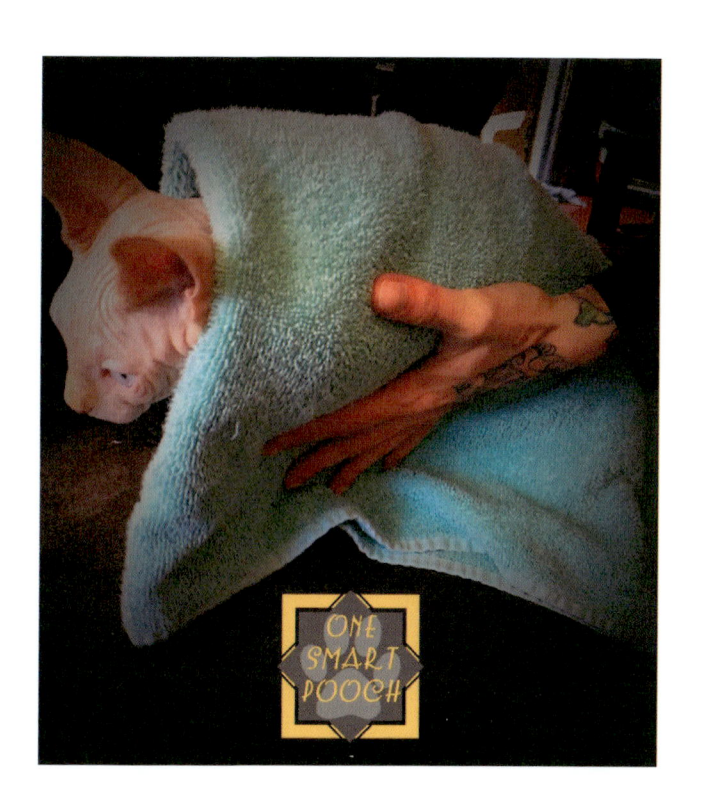

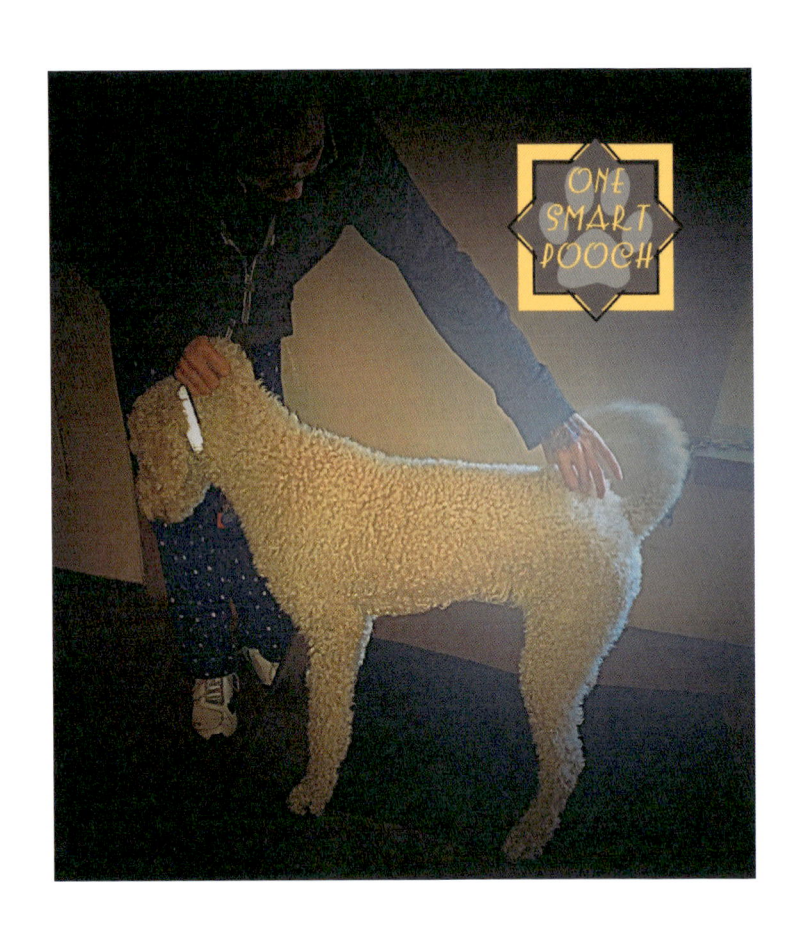

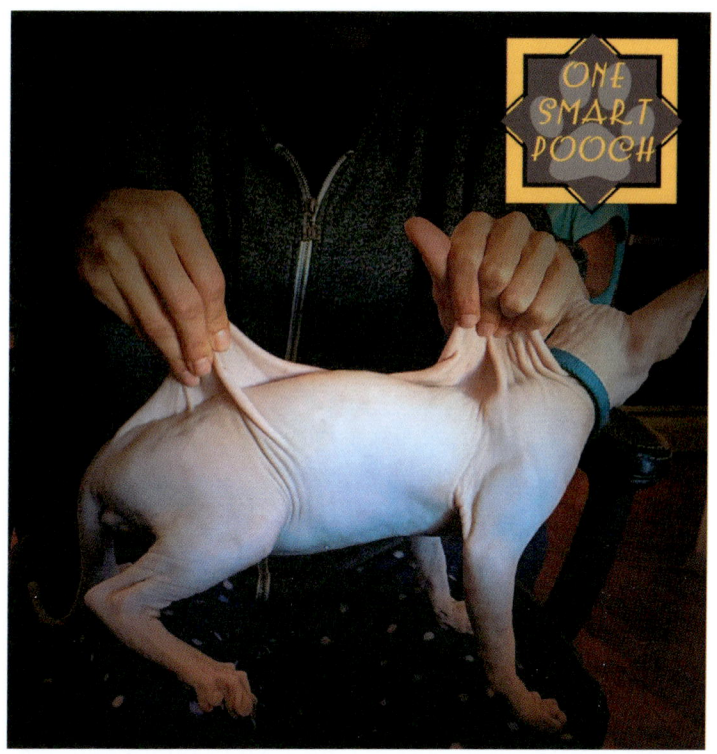

Note: If you hold the scruff too far down towards the shoulders your pet could turn his/her head to bite you.
~With your other hand, hold the back legs to restrain your pet.

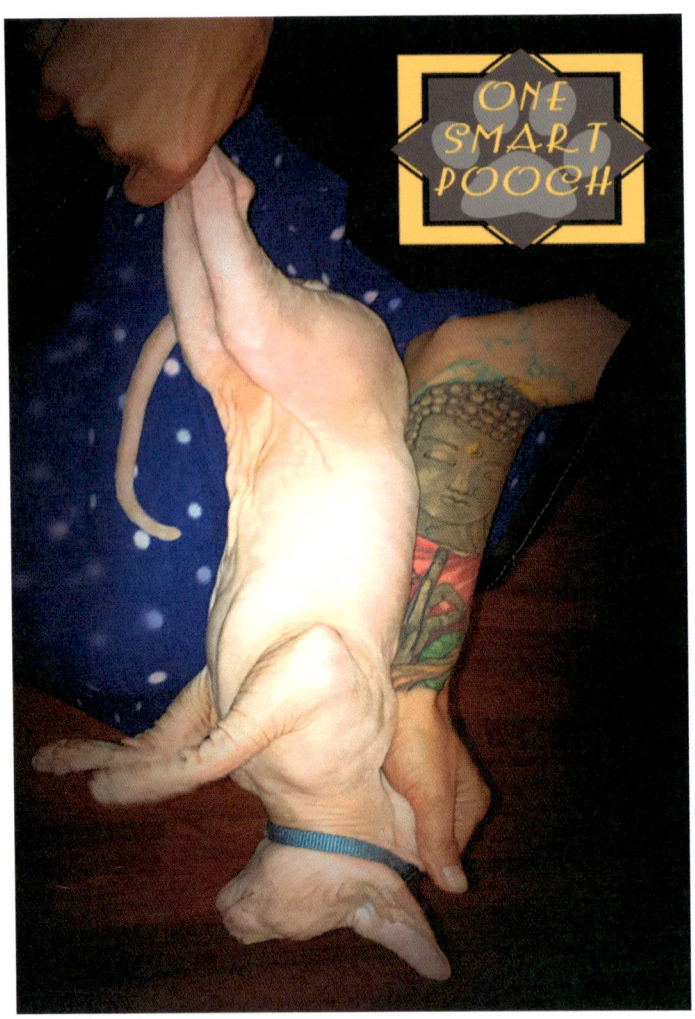

Temporary Muzzle
A temporary muzzle can be made by using a piece of soft cloth or a roll of gauze.
How to make a temporary muzzle out of a piece of soft cloth:
1. Make a loop in the center of fabric strip.
2. Slip loop over your pet's snout and tighten to firmly shut mouth.
Make sure fabric does not cut into your pet's skin!
3. Cross ends of fabric under chin exchanging ends in each hand.
4. Bring ends of fabric around each side of your pet's neck and tie off in a bow behind the ears.

ONE SMART POOCH

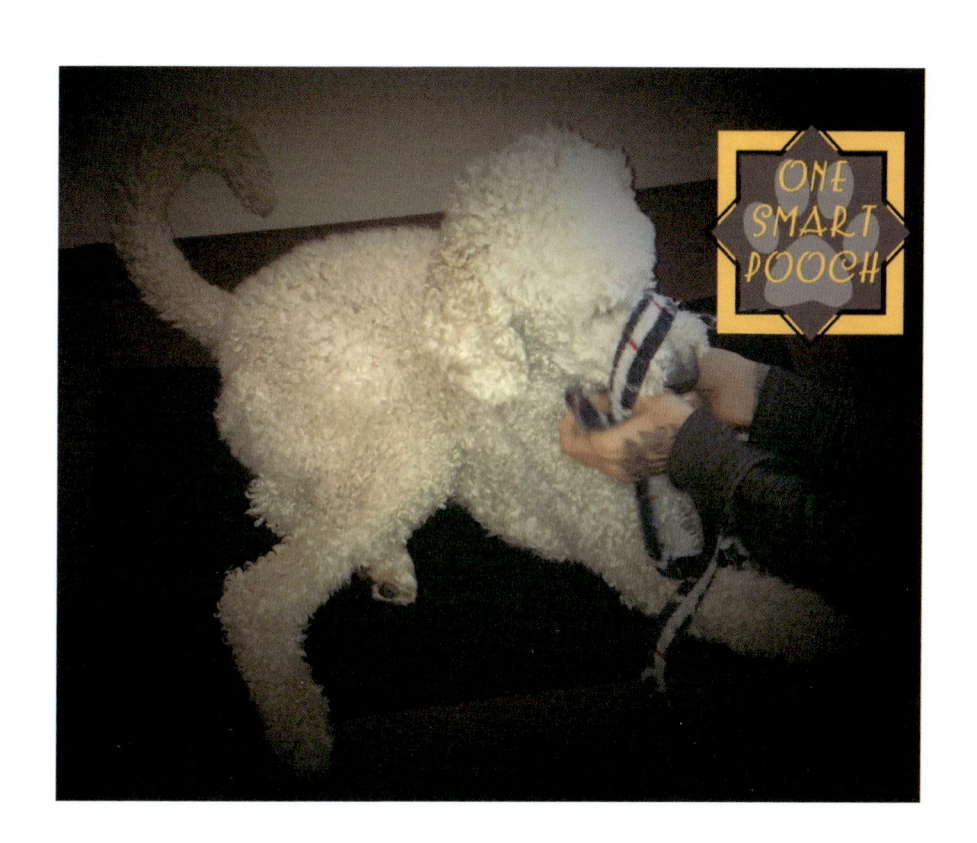

ONE SMART POOCH

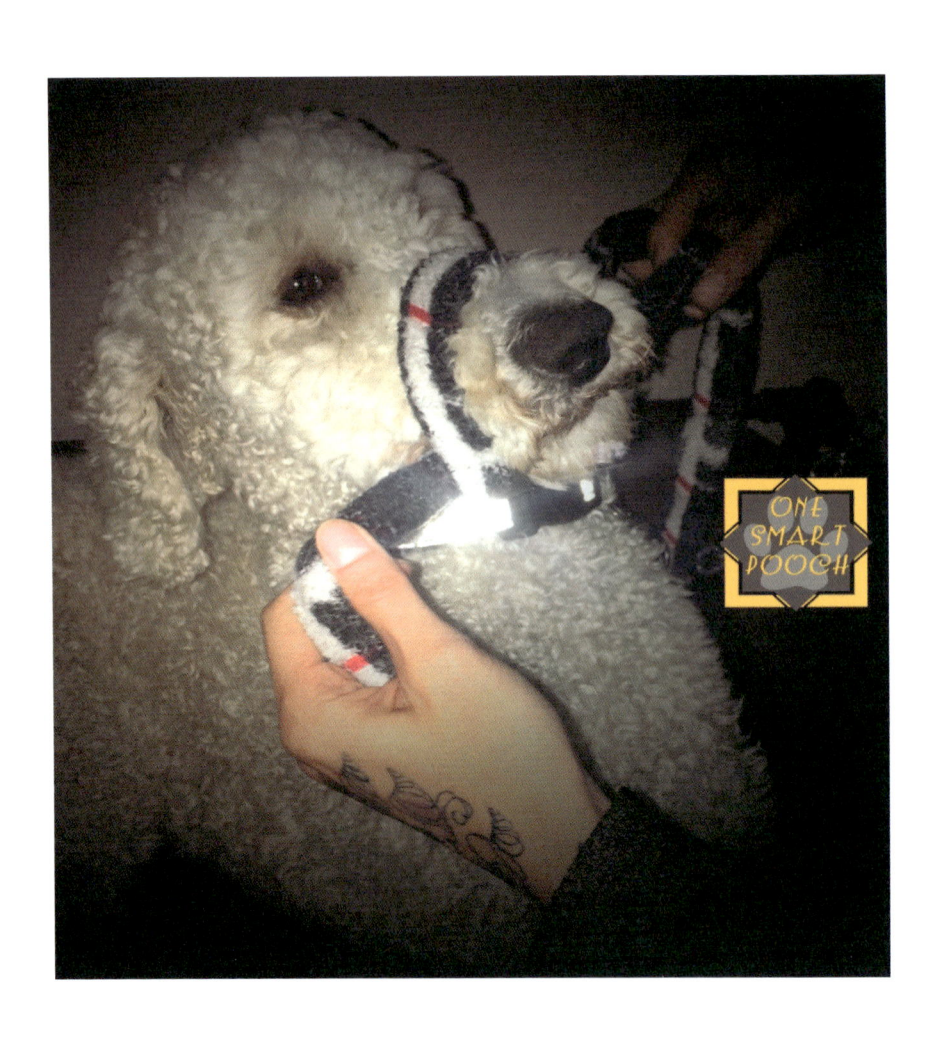

ONE SMART POOCH

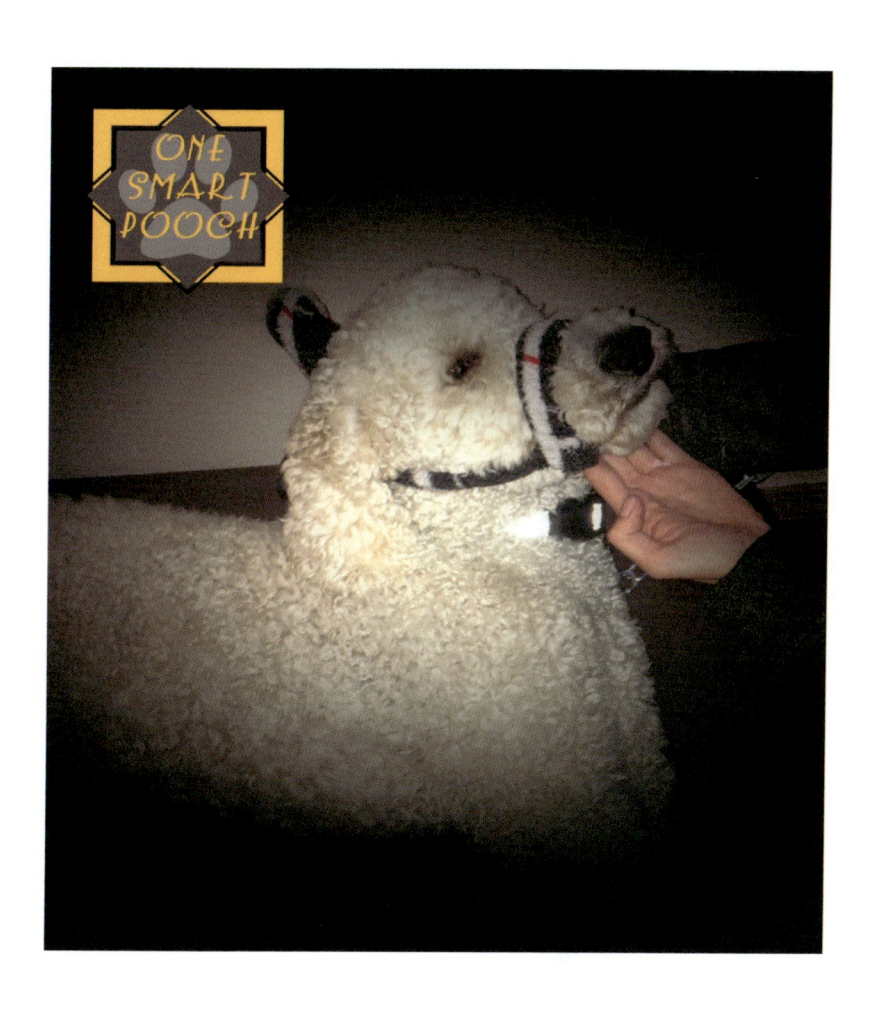

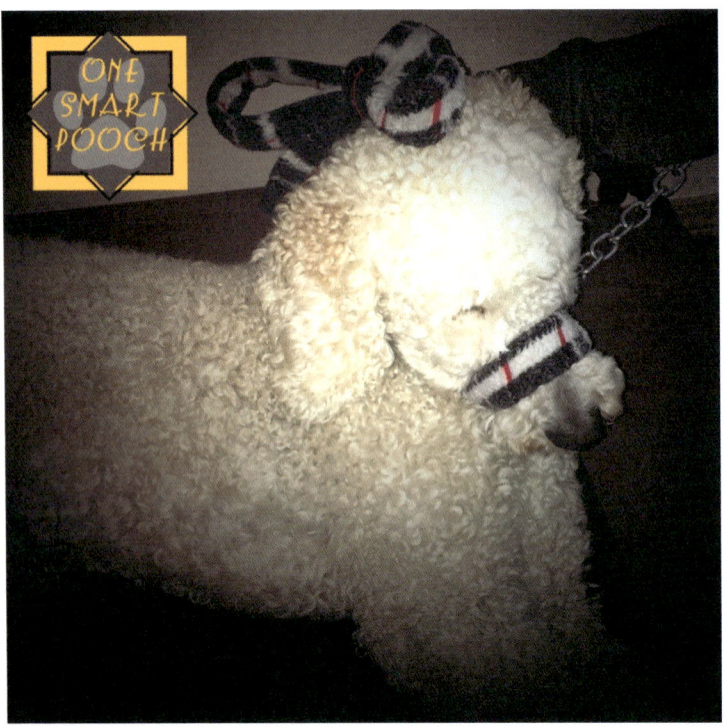

Never tie a knot!
Notes: Never leave a muzzled pet unattended!
If your pet is experiencing breathing difficulty, vomiting and/or seizures, do *NOT use a* muzzle because your pet could easily suffocate!
Fun Facts: Canines tend to have a den mentality and may even try to go hide to lick their wounds.
Felines when injured may try to fight or flee.

How to Transport & Carry your Injured or Sick Pet

~A towel can be place under the abdomen in front of your pet's hind legs as a sling to support a medium or large pet's hindquarters to assist him/her with walking.

~For an immobile pet you can make a makeshift stretcher by carefully sliding a towel underneath your pet. With the aid of another person holding one side, hold the sides taut and carry your pet to safety.

Note: If you happen to be alone with a large pet too big to carry, use the same method as above to drag your pet closer to help or transportation.

~Boards of many kinds can be used as backboards if you suspect your pet has a back and/or neck.

~For pets remove the top of a carrier/kennel or place your pet in a sturdy/strong cardboard box with the top open.
Note: Do *NOT* attempt to carry any pet on any backboard device if the animal is struggling or resisting restraint, this could cause more injuries.

Pet First-Aid Kits
Don't wasted time looking for items, be ready!

When you need to bandage a wound or even soothe an upset tummy, make sure you have everything you'll need in one spot, your Pet First-Aid Kit!

Pet first-aid kits should include:
- 4 X 4 gauze squares - used to control bleeding
- Rolled gauze - used to secure gauze squares in place, bandage a wound or to even make a temporary muzzle
- Adhesive tape or self-adhering bandage such as Vet-wrap→ - used to secure rolled gauze in place.
- Styptic powder and cotton swabs - used to control minor bleeding
- Bandage scissors or blunt-nose scissors - used to carefully remove bandages, cut proper lengths of bandaging materials or safely trim your pet's fur
- Tweezers - used to pull ticks or remove debris from a wound
- Hydrogen Peroxide (3%) - used to induce vomiting or clean an open wound
- Eye wash or sterile saline solution - used to flush minor wounds and clean eyes
- Chlorhexidine such as Hibiclens Liquid→ - used to flush cuts and wounds
- Cold pack - used to aid in Heat Stroke, swollen joints, burns and even bee stings
   Apply to injury removing frequently to prevent frostbite!
- Antibiotic ointment or diluted 15% tea tree oil or vitamin E gel or pure aloe-vera gel or Coconut oil - used to soothe and promote healing to open wounds, burns, or bee stings
   Apply externally to minor cuts, scrapes and insect bites.
  Notes: Do *NOT* use on animal bites, always see a Veterinarian for animal bites other than insects! If you use medical ointments instead of natural oil, make sure your pet can't lick the area and/or ingest the ointment.
- Needle-less dose syringe or eye dropper - used to administer medications and/or other liquids

- Digital thermometer - used to check your pet's temperature
- Antihistamine tablets such as Diphenhydramine or Benadryl→ - used for bee stings or allergic reactions
- Antacid tablets - used to soothe an upset stomach
- Electrolyte solution such as K9 Quencher→ or Pedialyte→ - used to aid in re-hydration
   Note: Sports-type drinks such as Gatorade are *NOT* recommended!
- Nylon slip-leash - used to restrain your pet
   Note: Can also be used as a temporary muzzle.
- Towel or blanket - used to treat for Shock and/or help transport your pet
   Notes: Can be used to cover your pet to maintain body heat and/or elevate his/her hindquarters to promote blood and air circulation. May also be used as a temporary stretcher and/or even as a sling to aid in walking.
- Pet First-Aid handbook - used to assist with important information you need to know
- Important names and phone numbers - pertaining information regarding your Veterinarian, nearest veterinary emergency center and animal poison control, readily available

How to Handle a Choking Pet

Signs of a Choking

- Loud noise or cough as an animal exhales
- Rasping noise as he inhales
- Gagging or retching as if trying to vomit
- Pawing at the mouth
- Drooling
- Outward stretching of the neck
- Staggering and eventually rapid/shallow breathing
- Pale/blue gums
- Collapse

Make sure you can see inside your pet's mouth, if you can see the object, carefully sweep in the mouth with your fingers (in the shape of a hook) to dislodge the object.

Try a technique below:

1) Place small pet on his/her stomach, in your lap, and lower his head in front of your knees. With the palm of your hand, deliver a firm blow, between the shoulder blades.

2) Stand behind your pet and place your arms around his/her waist. Close your hand making a fist, place your fist in the soft part of the stomach just behind the last rib, grasp the fist with your other hand, and compress the abdomen with 5 quick thrusts.

3) Place your hands or several fingers on each side of your pet's chest and thrust inward. After 2 to 3 thrusts, give him/her a moment to cough. Look in your pet's mouth, if you do not see the object, repeat.

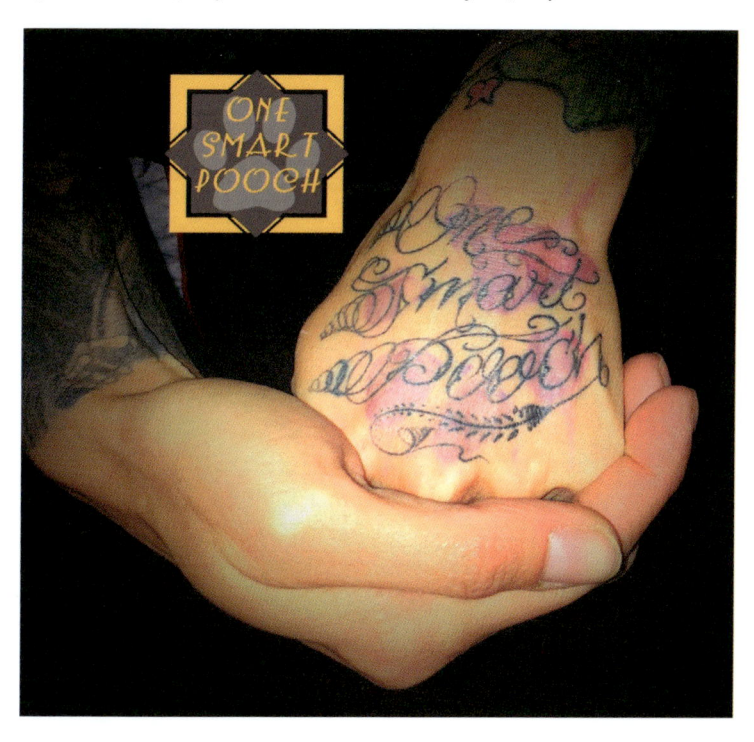

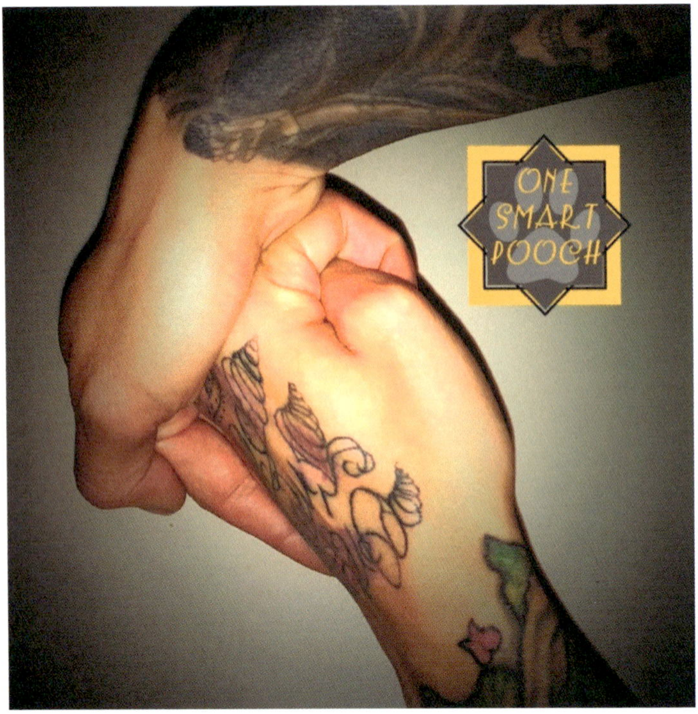
ONE SMART POOCH

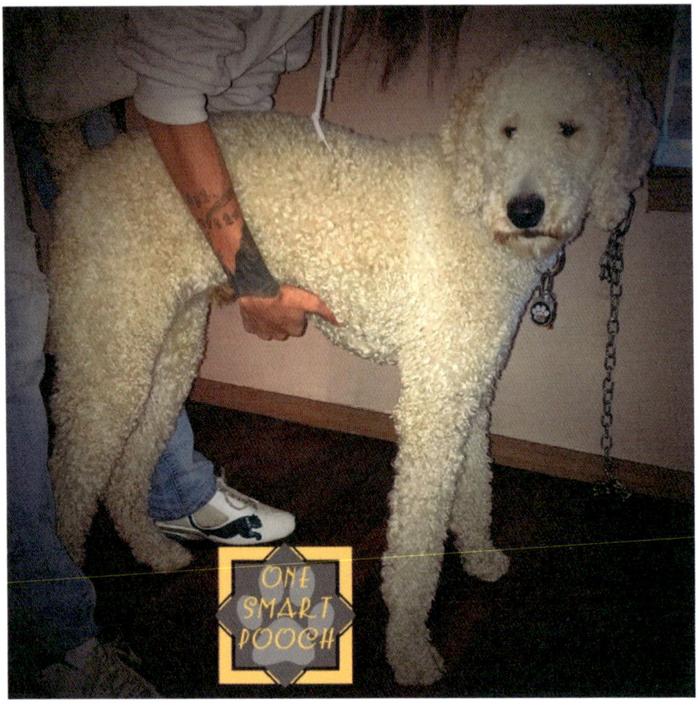
ONE SMART POOCH

Unconscious & Choking

Place your pet on his/her side and thrust with hand over hand on just one side of chest to squeeze the lungs.

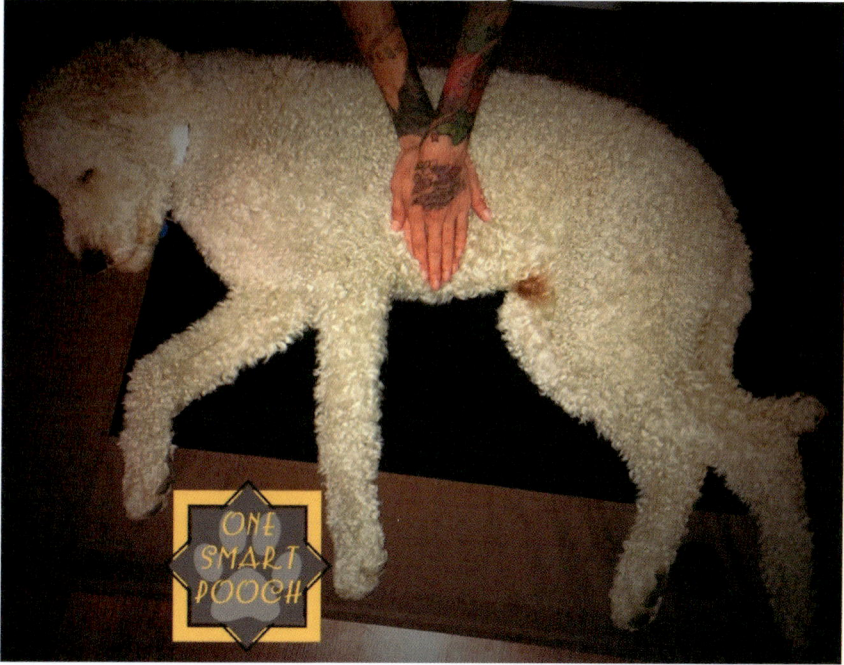

Alternate these thrusts, as described above, with Rescue Breathing & CPR, as described below.

Get to your veterinarian immediately!

Rescue Breathing plus CPR

Cardio Pulmonary Resuscitation (CPR) is the method of artificial life support.

A faster more efficient method is called *Cardio Pulmonary Cerebral Resuscitation* (CPCR).

Both techniques utilize a combination of chest compressions and artificial respirations. CPCR just focuses more on chest compressions and less on artificial respirations compared to CPR. CPCR utilizes the theory that the action of compressing the chest facilitates the movement of oxygen through the lungs, lessening the need for the administration of breaths through the nasal passage. Use 30 to 100 or more vigorous chest compressions between the administrations of Rescue Breathing.

Note: CPCR is used in cases when your pet has lost consciousness and/or both heartbeat and breathing are *NOT* detected.

CPR uses a combination of two hand positions for chest thrusts on small pets, hand position for chest thrusts for unconscious pets to ten compressions and the administration of one breath.
Emergency situations where CPCR may be required:

- Smoke Inhalation

- Heat Stroke or hyperthermia - Heat stroke internals an body temperature of 106.0 F or higher

- Electrocution

- Hit by Car

- Drowning

- Poisoning

- Choking

- Gunshot

- Hypoglycemia or low blood sugar

Remember: Even under the best of circumstances or in an animal ER with trained and experienced staff, medications, access to oxygen, tracheal tubes and IV catheters the outcome may *not* always be successful!
You will never know the outcome unless you try!

Fact: In an animal hospital setting only 4% of canines and 9.6% of felines successfully resuscitated via CPCR or CPR methods. According to the American Heart Association a human survival rate ranges from 6.4% - 20%.

Although you may have taken a human CPCR course, canines and felines don't share our anatomy. The concept of human and animal CPCR is the same with a different technique.

Below are the latest guidelines established by the North American Veterinary Conference or NAVC in 2011.

The ABC's or airway, breathing, circulation of CPR, known as CAB. American Heart Association have shown that keeping the blood flowing to the brain known as *circulation* is more valuable as a life-saving tool than the administration of artificial respiration.

The newest recommended protocol is CAB.

CAB = CIRCULATION, AIRWAY, BREATHING

Fun Fact: Veterinary communities all over have also adopted this protocol recommend by the American Heart Association.

Performing Rescue Breathing

- Rescue breathing in pets is done via the nasal passage.
- Make sure the pet's mouth is adequately closed and sealed.
- Evaluate the size your pet to judge the amount of artificial breaths you'll need to give.

It's *important* that you do NOT over-inflate your pet's lungs!

Rescue Breathing Technique

~With your pet on his/her side, gently close his/her mouth with one or two hands until his/her mouth is sealed.

Note: For a small pet, you may just need to use your thumb and index finger to make this seal.

- Close your hands around your pet's nose and create a tube-like space between the nose and your mouth avoiding direct contact with your pet's snout.
- Deliver two slow full breaths into your pet's nostrils.

Note: Make sure you see your pet's lungs rise and allow time for exhalation or see his/her lungs fall between the breaths.

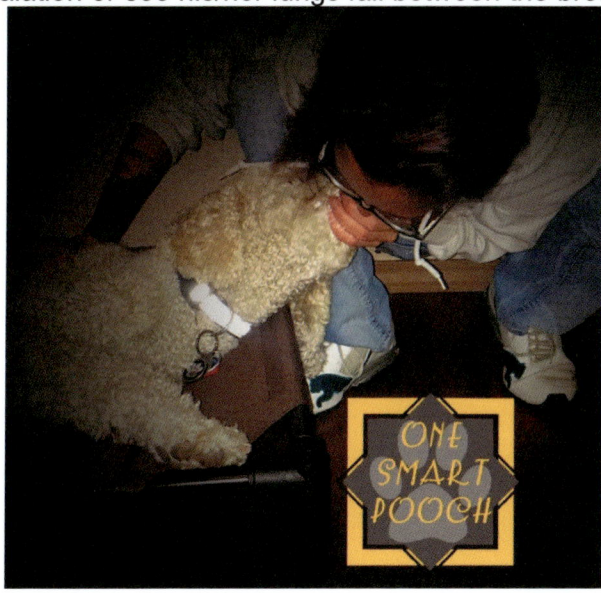

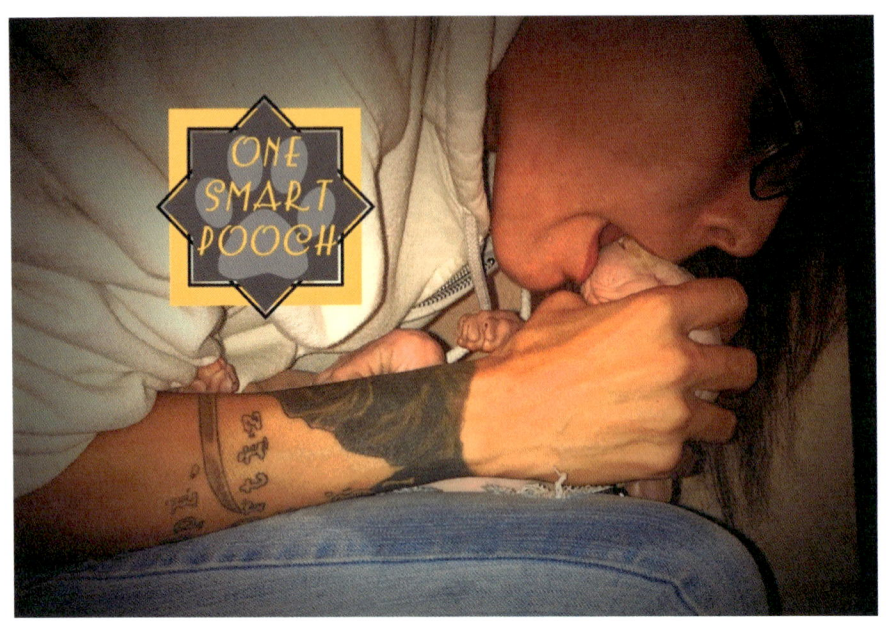

Performing CPCR

- Place your pet on the floor or a flat surface on his/her side and slightly extend head by pulling back on the chin to stretch out his/her throat.
- Take your pet's front legs, gently bending them at the elbow and bring them towards your pet's chest.

Note: Where the elbow touches your pet's chest is the proper place for your hands for compressions.

- Compress approximately 1/3 the width of your pet's chest diameter.
- When giving breaths, use your hands to seal off your pet's mouth and breathe directly into his/her nostrils.

Note: Use small puff like breathes, *ONLY*!

CPCR Technique

Never perform CPCR or rescue breathing on a conscious pet!

Medium to large size pet's more than three months of age:

1. Place your pet on the floor or a solid surface with their right side facing down.
2. Start chest compressions, 30 compressions.
3. Follow the compressions with 2 breaths into your pet's nostrils.
4. Repeat compressions, 30 compressions.

Note: Do *NOT* check your pet's status any sooner than 2 minutes, unless there's visible sign of recovery!

Tip: Theory is *"fast and hard"* to do the job!
For small pets less than three months of age:
~Follow above CPCR technique but place their chest in the palm of your hand or along your leg in your lap.
~Four fingers should be on one side of your pet, your thumb on the other side of the chest. Gently squeeze your fingers together to compress your pet's chest.

Note: The number of compressions should increase to 50 compressions per minute, followed by the administration of two breaths.

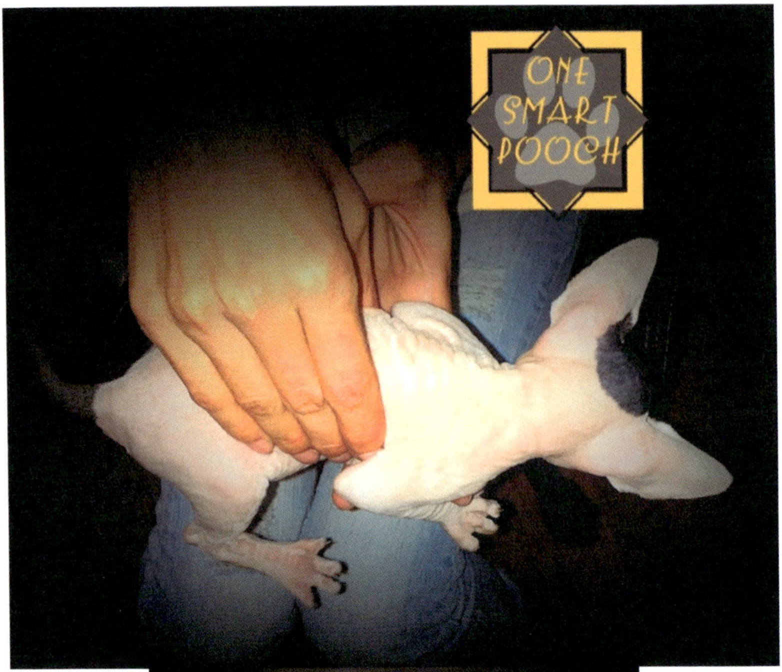

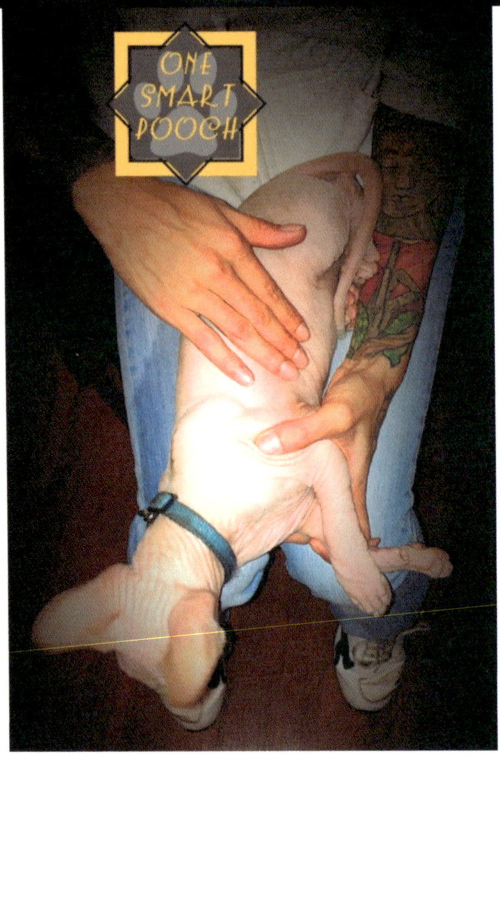

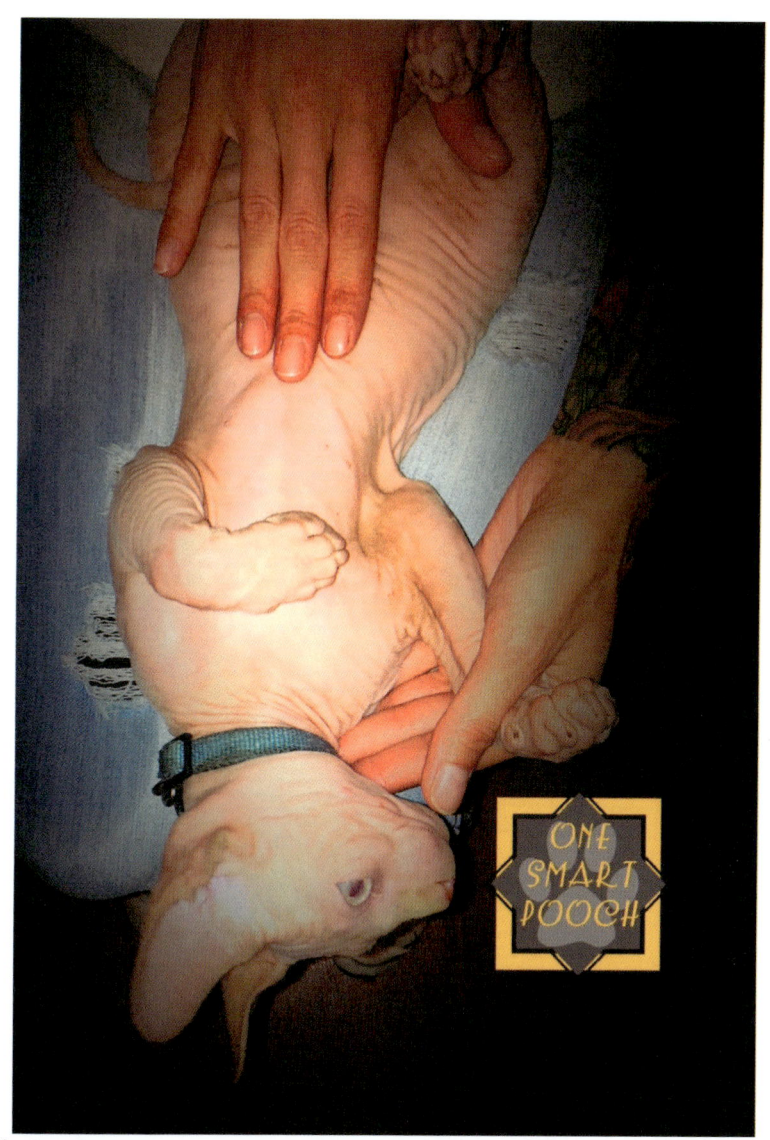

Note: Small and young pets do *NOT* require as much pressure during chest compressions!

For newborn puppies and kittens
Follow the same CPCR technique for small pets.
~Administer 1 compression and 1 puff breath at a time.
Note: If your hand covers your pet's entire torso, place your thumb on one-side of the chest and use only two fingers your index finger and middle finger on the other side.
~Gently squeeze your pet's chest with of your fingers.

Note: Rapid initiation of CPCR is critical.
Quickly transport your pet to the nearest animal emergency veterinary hospital!
You may not get your pet to breathe or resume a heart beat on his/her own and may even need to continue CPCR while someone else drives you to the nearest emergency veterinary hospital.
Do *NOT* stop administering CPCR until your pet shows signs of recovery or until a licensed veterinary can take over!
Facts: CPCR must be started within 4 minutes after the heart stops beating to avoid brain damage.
If the brain does not receive oxygenated blood within 10 minutes, brain damage is irreversible.

Basic First-Aid Techniques

Again, first-aid is *NOT* intended to replace your licensed veterinary care!
Your first responsibility is to ensure your *own* safety!
Do *NOT* attempt any first-aid techniques if it will pose any threat to your own health!

Birthing Difficulties or Dystocia

Pregnancy in canines and felines lasts approximately 63 days or between 60 to 65 days.

A common part of prenatal care is an x-ray after the 42_{nd} day of pregnancy to determine the number of neonates or fetuses the mother is carrying.

If a pregnancy lasts longer than 67 days see your licensed veterinary immediately!

Note: It's normal for bloody vaginal discharge to be present, up to 4 weeks after birth.

Signs your pet is near delivery:

- Mammary gland enlargement and milk secretion - 1 to 2 weeks prior to delivery
- Restlessness, seeking seclusion, anorexia, nesting - 12 to 24 hours prior to delivery
- Temperature decreases less than 99F - 8 to 24 hours prior to delivery

During the final stages, the fetuses or babies will begin to move through the birth canal.

Note: Your pet will experience obvious straining and involuntary contraction of the abdominal muscles.

Fun Fact: The brachycephalic breeds like Bull Dogs and Pekingese, are born with large heads and broad shoulders which could make it difficult for them to fit through their mother's pelvic canal making them prone to difficult deliveries and are more likely to require surgical intervention.

<u>Situations When You Should Offer Your Pet Some Assistance</u>
- If the neonate/fetus comes out only part of the way despite the mother's efforts!

~To assist, gently grasp the emerging puppy or kitten with a clean washcloth and gently pull him/her free.

Note: Do *NOT* attempt to remove a neonate/fetus or baby if you cannot see both the front legs and head!

- If the mother doesn't instinctively tear off the amniotic sac within 30 seconds.

~Carefully and gently peel away the amniotic sac from around the baby's face.

~Clean the mucus from the baby's mouth with your finger and then rub the newborn vigorously with a clean cloth until you hear the newborn cry or make a noise.

~Encourage the mother to lick her young and sever/eat the umbilical cord.

- If the mother does *NOT* sever/eat the umbilical cord within one minute.

~Severing the umbilical cord for the mother by tying two pieces of embroidery thread around the umbilical cord.

Notes: The first thread should be tied about 1 ½ inches from the tummy.
The second thread should be tied about an inch farther down the umbilical cord from the first thread you tied.

~Clean a pair of sharp bandage scissors with rubbing alcohol.

~Then snip or cut the umbilical cord between the two threads you tied.

<u>Signs of a life-threatening emergency</u>
- The mother passes dark green fluid called lochia before the birth of the first baby.

Note: This could mean the placenta has separated prematurely.

- The mother has been straining consonantly without delivering a young for more than an hour.

Note: This could mean that the baby is too large or may even be in the wrong position to pass through the mother's birth canal.

- If the mother appears weak, nervous or restless for more than a half hour after the major labor signs have stopped.
Note: This could mean there's still be another baby stuck inside the mother's birth canal.
- If the mother experiences muscle tremors days or weeks after giving birth, begins to vomit and/or has any troubles standing.
Note: These may be signs of Eclampsia.
Eclampsia is a life threatening calcium deficiency that can occur after a mother gives birth.

Bleeding

Arterial bleeding is of the utmost urgency!
The largest vessels carrying blood and oxygen throughout your pet's body is known as the Arteries.
Arterial blood will appear bright red due to oxygen saturation.

<u>A severed artery can result in:</u>
- Large amounts of quick blood lost
- Spurting blood as the arterial blood pumps blood directly from your pet's heart
Note: Injury to a vein, another large blood vessel, could also result in massive blood loss.

<u>Differences in an arterial bleeding and vein bleeding include:</u>
- Darker blood because as it travels through the body it picks up toxins along the way
- Steady stream of bleeding
Note: A situation like this will require you to flush out the wound to help prevent any kind of infections!

<u>Minor cuts and scrapes:</u>
- Flush with water, saline solution, eye wash and/or Chlorhexidine
Note: If your pet starts to lick at his/her wound, bandage loosely and/or apply a cone collar on the animal.
- Use styptic powder or baking flower to control bleeding toenails
Note: Watch to make sure your pet's injury doesn't become infected.

<u>Severe bleeding injuries to the legs or limbs:</u>
- Apply direct pressure with gauze pads or clean towel over the wound to stop the bleeding
- If the limb has *not* stopped bleeding after a few minutes of pressure, elevate the limb that is bleeding by placing a pillow or folded towel under the injured limb
Note: Try to elevate above your pet's heart.

- If above steps do *not* work to control the bleeding; apply pressure to one of the 5 arterial pressure points to diminish blood flow
    Note: The pressure points are located in areas where your pet's arteries are closest to the surface of his/her skin.

<u>Pressure Point Locations:</u>
*The front leg, above the elbow joint, toward the inside of the front leg, in your pet's armpit area

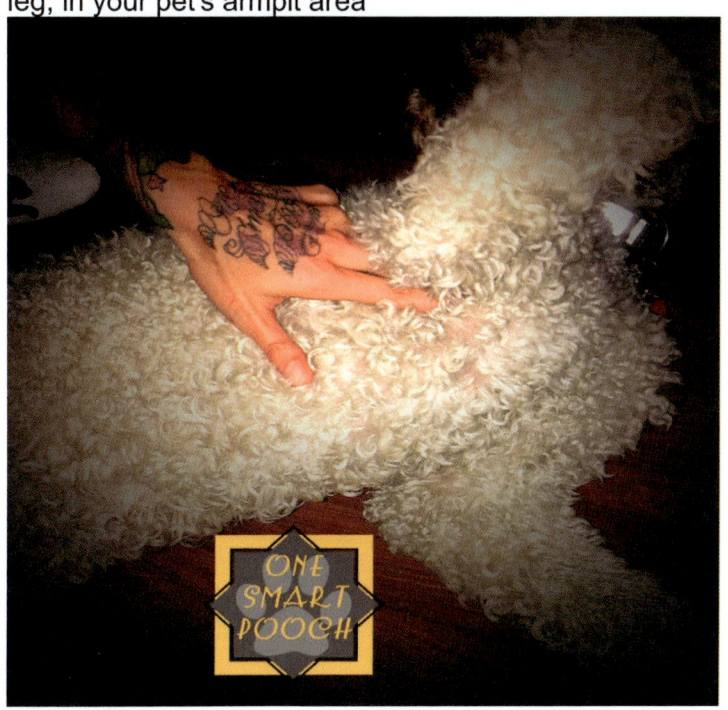

*The rear leg, on the inside of your pet's upper thigh, where his/her leg meets the body

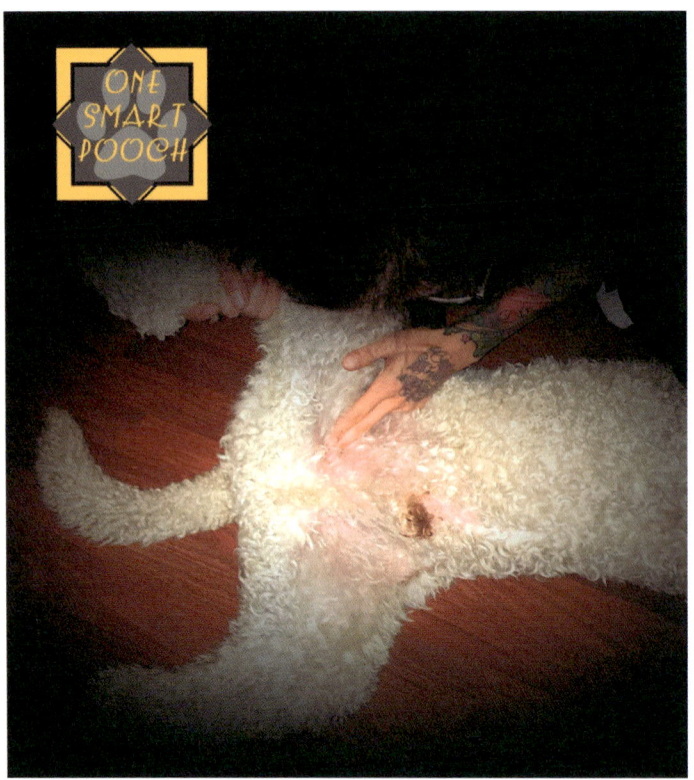

*The front foot, behind your pet's front foot, just above his/her largest pad

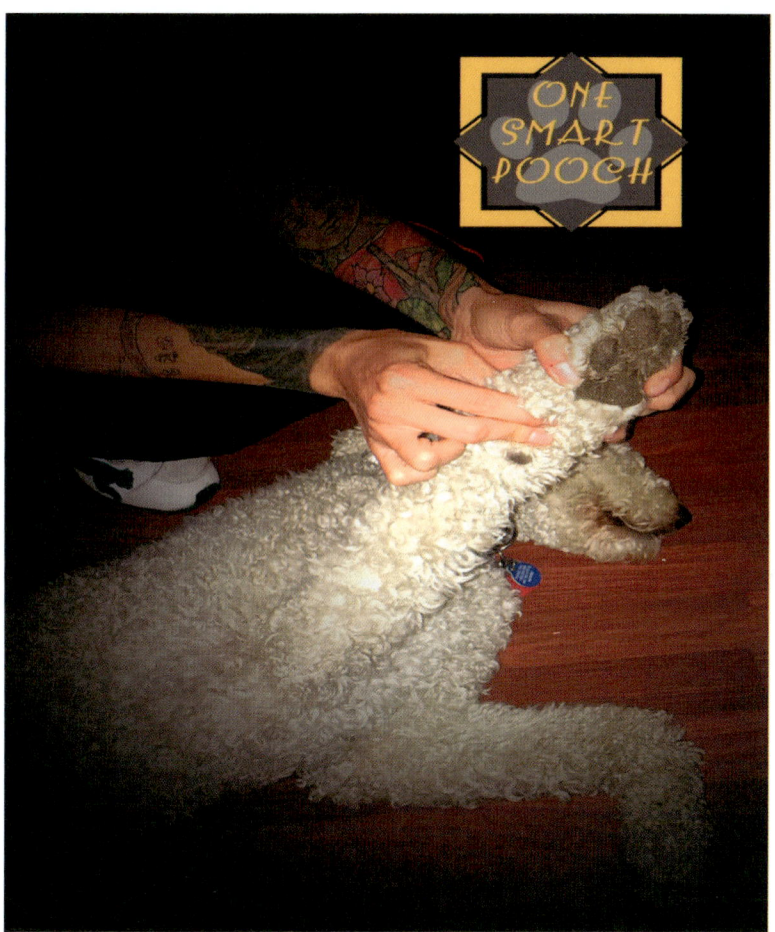

*Behind your pet's rear foot, just above his/her largest pad

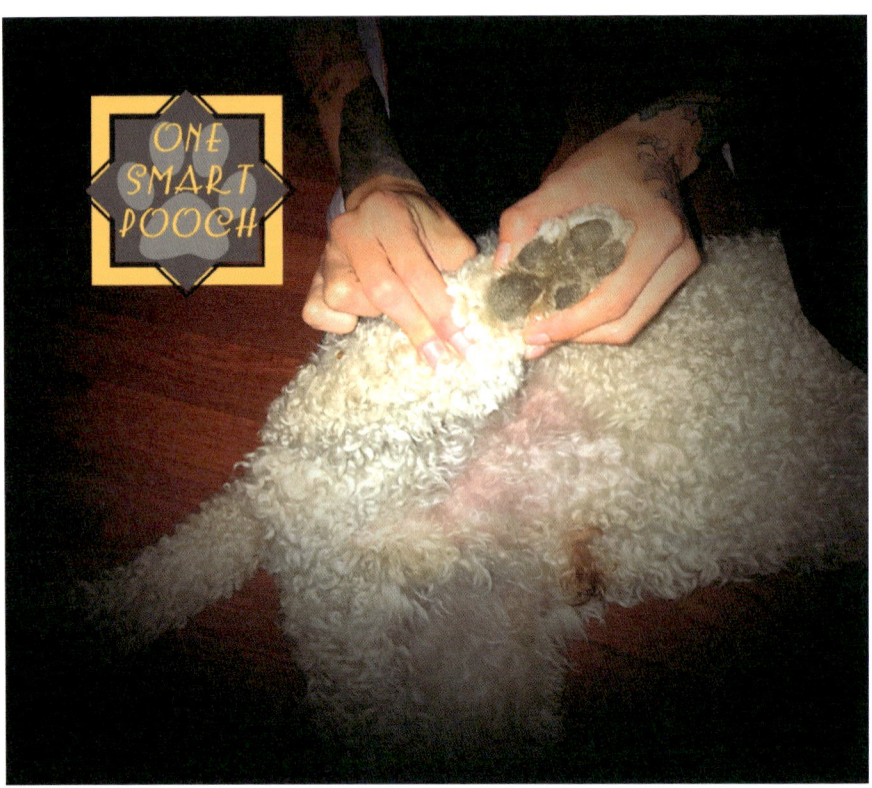

*The underside of your pet's tail, at the base

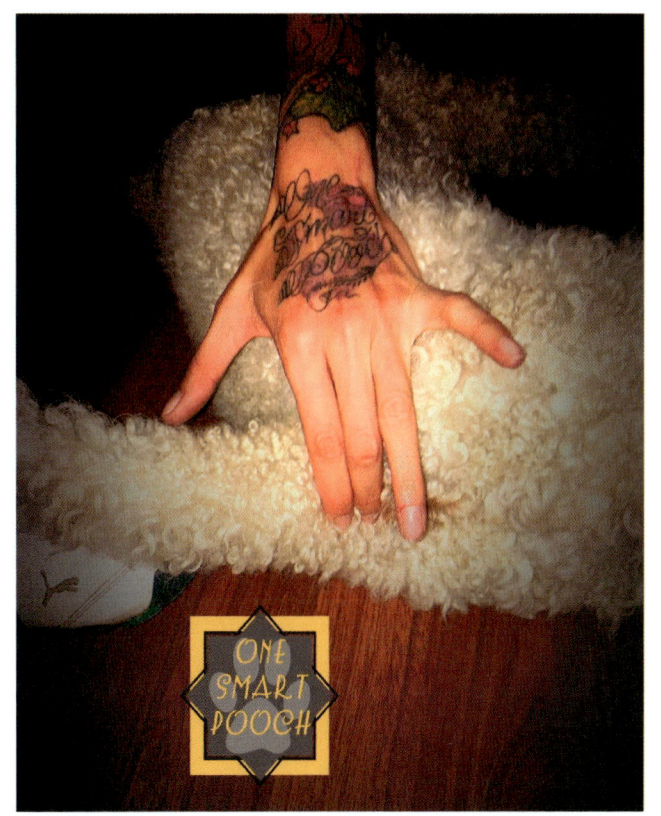

Note: Pick the pressure point that is in direct correlation or close to your pet's injury!

• Wrap flat gauze with rolled gauze, overlapping each layer by about — widths each time around the leg, then secure with self-adhering elastic bandage making sure you can slip a finger underneath, then get to your licensed veterinarian for help!

  Note: Never apply a tourniquet to control severe bleeding!

Paw Pad Wounds

• Remove obvious debris and/or flush the pads clean.
• Elevate if needed to control the bleeding.
• Dry the paw pad and bandage by placing a non-stick pad on the wound.
• In a figure eight pattern, wrap your pet's paw pad with gauze going between each of the toes to hold it in place.

  Note: Secure firmly. But, *NOT* too tightly!

Ear Injuries

• If your pet's ears are higher than the heart already, you already have built-in/natural elevation.

- Press upright ears down against your pet's cheek to apply direct pressure, if the ear's bleeding.
- Flip your pet's ear downward, up and fold onto the top of head to apply direct pressure.
- Bandage your pet's ear in place using the good ear as an anchor by going around the good ear first, then back behind the ear to secure the ear in place.
- Use the sleeve off a cotton t-shirt or cut the toe off a cotton sock and use it like a headband, over the ears to hold the bandage in place.

Note: For small cuts, styptic powder or baking flower may be used to control bleeding.

Tail Injuries

- Apply direct pressure with a gauze pad and lift your pet's tail to elevate.
- If you have to, press on the pressure point at base of your pet's tail to diminish blood flow.
- Wrap your pet's tail up with gauze. Then slip a cotton sock over the gauze wrap.
- Beginning at the tip of your pet's tail, wrap sock in a figure-eight pattern with adhesive tape going up his/her tail.
- Complete the figure-eight back down your pet's tail.

Note: Be careful *not* to wrap too tightly!

Chest Injuries

- Apply direct pressure with gauze, directly over the chest wound.
- There are no applicable pressure points in your pet's chest area.
- When applying a gauze roll, wrap it around your pet's entire torso to hold it in place, and then secure it to itself with adhesive tape.

Notes: An alternative could be, fit your pet in a child size cotton t-shirt or socks with holes in the toes.

If the bleeding does *NOT* stop within 15 minutes after applying direct pressure, seek veterinary care immediately!

Burns

Felines love heat and will lounge on surfaces well over 100.0 F. They are even attracted to gas stoves and/or sometimes candles. Canines on the other hand, will usually shy away from heat.
Our pets can obtain first, second, and third degree burns. Plus, tissue damage from chemicals and/or electrical sources.

Depending on the severity of the burn, a visit to your licensed Veterinarian may be required!

But, before going to the Vet, your primary goal is to stop *the cooking or constant burning* of your pet's skin and tissues. Alongside, alleviating discomfort, which can range from being uncomfortable to intense pain.

Remember to safely restrain your pet before assisting in any aid!

First Degree Burns, caused by a heat source such as a gas stove – skin appears dark pink/red

- Your first goal is to cool the skin down with room temperature water

   Note: Do *NOT* apply ice to a burn it can restrict your pet's blood flow!

- Carefully trimming your pet's fur away from the burn with blunt-nosed scissors and apply pure aloe-vera gel to promote healing

   Note: If your pet's skin is broken/open see your licensed Veterinarian!

   Facts: First degree burn is most commonly caused by sunburn. First degree burn is the least-severe type of burn.

Second Degree Burns, caused by a heat source such as an electric stove top – blisters and/or fluids, clear fluid (commonly found in blisters) is present

- Flush the burn gently with cool water for 5-10 minutes

   Note: NOT ice-cold water!

- Pat dry with a soft cloth or paper towel

   Note: Do *NOT* use cotton balls, cotton swabs, or toilet paper!

- Bandage loosely, using a non-stick pad, and ace bandage wrap
- Then see your veterinarian for help immediately!

   Note: Do *NOT* apply any kind of gels, ointments or sprays! Medications are best determined and prescribed by your licensed veterinarian!

   Facts: Second degree burns are painful for our pets and are susceptible to infection since there are open sores.

Second degree burns may continue to cause damage and burn even after the initial source of the burn has been removed or flushed away.

The flow of cool water reduces your pet's temperature beneath the skin surface to help prevent further damage to the skin and/or tissue.

Third Degree Burns (caused by a heat source such as a hot frying pan) – skin will appear charred, white and/or a leathery and brown color

- Restrain your pet and bandage the burn loosely
- Do *NOT* apply any kind of gels, ointments and/or sprays
  Note: Medications are best determined and prescribed by your licensed veterinarian!
- Monitor your pet for signs of shock on the way to your veterinarian
  Fun Facts: Third degree burns goes through all layers of your pet's skin and even into their muscle underneath the skin. Third degree burns are more serever than second degree burn. Third degree burns are often less painful than second degree burns because they destroy the nerve endings in the burned area.
  Note: Third degree burns will always require immediate care from your licensed veterinarian!

Chemical Burns

- Flush liquid chemicals from your pet's body with cool to lukewarm water for about 10 minutes.
  Notes: Water that's too hot may speed up the absorption of the chemical through your pet's skin. Water that is too cold can cause your pet to go through hypothermia.
- If you believe your pet has been exposed to a chemical agent that may affect your pet's lungs, monitor his/her breathing for 24 to 48 hours.
  Note: If you notice abnormal breathing, see your veterinarian immediately!
- If chemical is oily or greasy like car oil and in your pet's fur or on his/her skin, put dishwashing liquid into your pet's fur/skin first to dissolve grease before flushing with water. Wash with dishwashing liquid to clean the fur and skin.
- If it's a dry chemical such as powdered or granular, brush away or even vacuum out your pet's fur if he/she will allow you to do so safely.
  Notes: Adding water could further activate the chemical, so do *NOT* flush with water until all the dry chemical has been removed. See your veterinarian immediately if the burn appears to be either second or third degree burns! Bring the chemical container with you to your veterinarian.

Electrical Burns

Do *NOT* touch your pet if he/she has been electrocuted until the electricity is turned off or the source of electrocution is safely away from both you and your pet!

- Immediately check to see if your pet is breathing and has a pulse
- If your pet is not breathing, administer Rescue Breathing or CPCR, if his/her heartbeat is also absent

Get to your veterinarian immediately!

- Check your pet for burns to his/her face or in their mouth
- Check for bite marks on any electrical cords or a burning odor in the room could imply your pet was burned or shocked

Notes: Even if your pet is conscious after electrocution, you should still see your veterinarian!

Even minor electrical shocks can damage blood vessels in your pet's lungs which could cause a leak of fluids that can make breathing difficult for your pet.

It could take anywhere from several hours to two days before symptoms such as shortness of breath, loss of appetite, and/or lethargy to set in.

Do *NOT* delay veterinary care from your veterinarian!

Drowning

~If you find your pet in a body of water, quickly remove him/her by pulling their collar with whatever stick or rod you can find.

~For larger pets, place in wheelbarrow position, front legs on ground while you hold up hind legs with care *NOT* to hit your pet's snout or head on the ground.

Note: Take care and do *NOT* try this on an aggressive, shy, or dominant pet!

~Hold felines and small canines securely by their hind legs to drain water from their lungs, windpipe and mouth. For large canines, lay your pet on his/her side and elevate hind quarters with cushions or a folded blanket to help drain water from their lungs, windpipe and mouth.

~With your pet on his/her side, it may help release water if you place the heel of your hand in the dip behind the last rib and thrust up towards your pet's head 3-4 times.

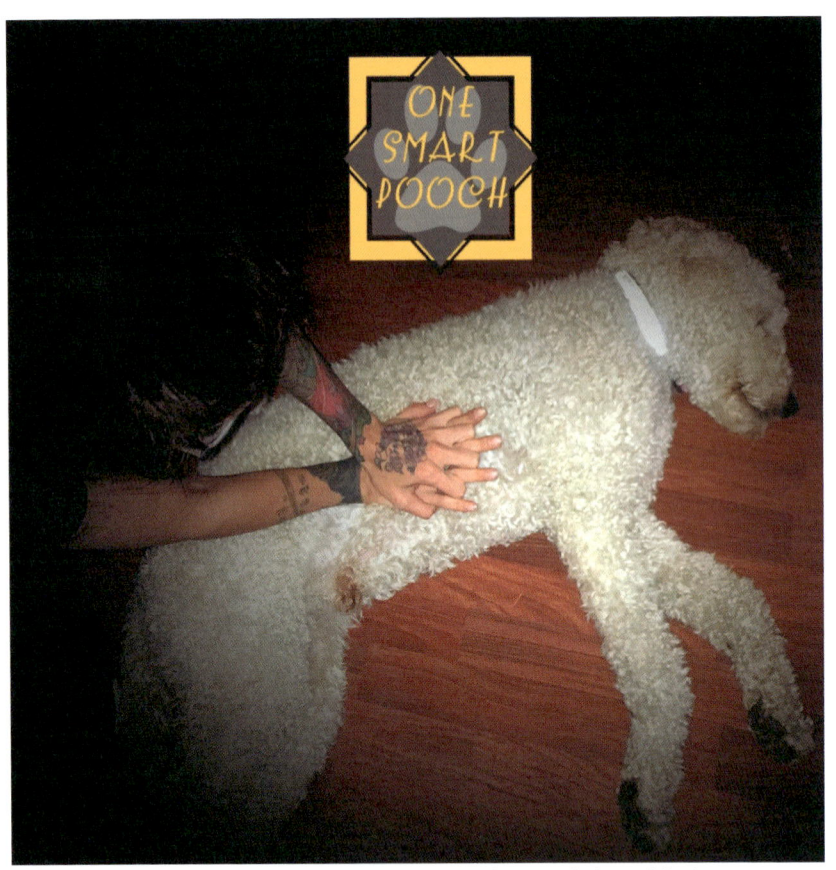

Note: Do *NOT* spend more than a minute doing this because your pet's lungs will quickly absorb water and any water that does not come out quickly probably won't come out at all!

~If there's a heartbeat but your pet is not breathing, begin rescue breathing immediately!

~Wrap your pet in a towel or blanket to keep from going into hypothermia and continue rescue breathing until your pet shows signs of breathing or until your licensed veterinarian can take over for you!

~If your pet is not breathing and has no heartbeat, begin CPCR and get prompt veterinary help.

Note: Do *NOT* stop CPCR unless your pet shows signs of recovery or until a licensed veterinarian can take over for you!

Fun Facts: Believe it or not, canines and felines do not know how to swim at birth; some do not know how to swim at all. Some canine breeds with short necks have difficulty keeping their heads above water while trying to swim.

Tip: Make any water environment safe for your pet by fencing it off, attaching a pet ramp to the side of your swimming pool or making your pet wear a life-jacket when at the lake or beach.

Falls and/or High-Rise Syndrome

Falling felines do *NOT* always land on their feet! Felines can sustain injuries like broken bones, broken jaws, ruptured organs and/or even death from falling out of open windows, off of balconies and even from trees.

Canines are just as likely to be injured in the event of a fall. They do not typically land on their feet like felines. A canine's body is typically heavier than a feline's body, meaning that they fall faster and harder, increasing the risk of injury.

Even if you don't see your pet fall, a limp or refusal to move and/or eat should alert you to a broken bone or even internal injuries.

If you witness your pet fall from any elevated area, check and do the following:

- First check to see if your pet is breathing and has a heartbeat.
  Note: If not, administer CPCR or rescue breathing and get to your licensed veterinarian immediately!
- If your pet is conscious, check for bleeding and internal injuries like broken bones and treat accordingly.
  Note: Any bleeding in the eyes, nose and/or mouth could mean your pet has a possible head injury!
- If your pet can't get up and/or refuses to get up he/she could have a back injury. Keep your pet as still as possible.
  Note: Do *NOT* try to pick your pet up to move him/her if a back or neck injury is suspected! Instead, slide a flat object like a cookie sheet or cutting board underneath him/her and then secure your pet with a towel or gauze.

Fun Facts: Felines have a fluid-filled organ in their inner ear called vestibular apparatus that helps them balance themselves out during a fall. In a study from the Journal of American Veterinary Medical Association, 132 felines were studied who had fallen out of high-rise windows. On average, the felines who fell 5 1/2 stories, 90% of the felines survived. Most suffered severe injuries. On high falls, the abdomen and chest absorbed more of the impact rather than their head and/or legs. During the shorter falls, felines often landed on their feet with their legs rigid, that resulted in multiple fractures, chest, jaw, bone, joint & spinal injuries, concussions and ruptures of internal organs.

The best cure for High-Rise Syndrome is prevention!

Tip: Make sure you have screens securely in place on all your windows and do not leave your pet unsupervised on balconies, rooftops or any other high places.

Frostbite

Canines and felines are *NOT* immune to extreme-weather ailments or changes such as 79°F one day the 50°F the next. Our pets can't tell us when their paws and/or feet are getting numb. We usually find out once it starts hurting them to step and/or the tissue is hard/frozen, frostbitten. If dark in color, generally surgery is required by your veterinarian.
~Promptly get your pet out of the cold and into a warmer environment.
~Wrap your pet's frozen paws with blankets or towels
Tip: Tumble towels or blankets briefly in a warm, *not* hot, clothes dryer.
Note: Do *NOT* massage the area if the tissue is hard, it will cause more pain!
~To promote circulation to your pet's frostbitten parts have your pet lay on your lap or on a sofa with his/her legs, paws, and tail, if affected, lowered.
See your licensed veterinarian immediately!

Heat Stroke

Pets left in a vehicle, shed, garage, etc. for a short period of time can be deadly for your pet in the summer heat.
Canines and Felines do *NOT* sweat to regulate their body temperatures like we do. They release body heat through their tongue, nose and pads. Canines pant to exchange cooler outside air with the warm humid air in their lungs. Felines do not normally pant until they are overwhelmed by the heat and/or overwhelmed with excited play. If the outside air is not cooler than your pet's body temperature, your pet could have a Heat Stroke.
Without immediate care a Heat Stroke can result in brain damage, kidney failure, cardiac arrest and/or even death. Older and/or overweight pets as well as short-nosed breeds like Pugs are at high risk for heat stroke.

Fun Fact: 100.0°F – 102.5°F is normal body temperature.
Symptoms of Heat Stroke may include:
- heavy panting
- gasping
- dehydration
- vomiting, *IF* not already dehydrated

- foaming at or around the mouth
- weak or high pulse
- inability to drink water
- bright red or suddenly bluish gums
- loss of consciousness

Heat Stroke is a life-threatening emergency condition that requires care from your licensed veterinarian!

If you suspect your pet is suffering from a Heat Stroke do the following:

- Move your pet to a cooler environment to prevent his/her internal body temperature from continuing to rise.

Tip: Indoors with a cool fan blowing on your pet, even a shady sidewalk or shady grassy area could help.

- Immerge your pet in lukewarm, *NOT* ice, water beginning with your pet's paws on up to his/her head and back. If your pet's too large and/or you don't have the appropriate size tub, getting the skin on his/her paws, pits, groin and belly wet will help cool your pet down.
- Rubbing alcohol applied with a wash cloth to your pet's inner flaps of his/her ears and pads will help cool your pet.

Note: Do *NOT* douse your pet with the rubbing alcohol or pour the rubbing alcohol on your pet! This could cause a sudden change in body temperature and result in shock!

- Placing a cool/ice pack or bag of frozen vegetables on your pet's neck to help him/her cool off.

Note: Remove the ice pack every 5 to 10 minutes to make sure you don't cause frostbite.

- Do *NOT* force your pet to drink water as he/she could aspirate water into their lungs.
- Check your pet's temperature and if it's 103.0°F or higher, get to your licensed Veterinarian immediately! Wrap your pet in a wet sheet or towel, turn on the car's air conditioning and drive quickly but safely to your veterinarian.
- If your pet goes unconscious, rub a little honey or Karo Syrup→ on his/her gums to increase blood sugar levels, and be ready to administer CPCR.
- If your pet temperature drops to 100°F, cover him/her with a blanket and place an 2-liter bottle filled with warm, *NOT* hot, water

next to him/her as you transport him/her to your licensed Veterinarian.

Hot Spots and/or Lick Sores

Felines seldom get hot spots, but canines can develop red, wet sores that make their skin look raw that can be caused by a wide range of things. The spots on their skin can begin to itch and cause your pet to lick and/or chew at it causing bacteria to grow and quickly spread creating a wound that can be very painful or could even get infection. Generally if the spot only involves the top layer of skin the spot can/could heal quickly with simple first-aid.

~Trim your pet's fur around the sore with blunt-nosed scissors so that you can easily clean the area with warm water.
~Gently pat the area dry with a soft wash cloth.
~Do *NOT* apply ointments to a hotspot as these products seal in infections and may burn!

Note: Instead use an antibacterial spray or cream that dries up/out the sore or apply a tea bag, black tea, *NOT* herbal tea, that has cooled after being soaked in hot water for 5 minutes.
Use this treatment 3-5 times a day until the spots are healed.
Hot spots that show no obvious signs of improvement for more than 7 days should be seen by your licensed veterinarian!

Embedded Object

If you find yourself in the unfortunate situation of finding your pet with a stick, arrow or other object imbedded into his/her body do the following:

• Keep your pet still.
• Secure the object in the exact position it's in by placing gauze rolls on both sides of the wound and then wrap with a third roll.
• Make the wrap snug enough to hold the object in place.

Note: *Not* tight enough to restrict your pet's blood flow or breathing!

• Place a brace around the embedded object by cutting a hole in the top of a Plastic or Styrofoam cup and put the object through the cup. Then with medical tape, tape the container firmly to your pet's body to prevent movement.
The split allows the object to penetrate up and through the container but will help the object to remain in place.

Note: Do *not* attempt to brace or stabilize an embedded object if your pet is struggling or showing obvious signs of extreme pain and/or aggression!
You could cause the object to become embedded further in to your pet's skin or cause more physical harm to your pet.

- Transport your pet to a licensed veterinarian hospital immediately!

Important Note: *NEVER* attempt to remove an embedded object that has punctured all layers of your pet's skin!
This could cause more severe bleeding and/or tissue/organ damage.

Vomiting and/or Diarrhea

Vomiting and diarrhea can/could be the result of poisoning or illnesses.

But, most of the time it's a simple digestive upset or upset stomach. Your pet may have eaten too much, too fast, they might have even eaten something that was spoiled and/or gotten into your garbage can.

If your pet is experiencing vomiting and/or diarrhea and you know it's *not* the result of poisoning do the following to help your pet:

- Rest your pet's stomach by withholding his/her food for 24 hours.

  Note: Always provide fresh water in small but frequent doses because if your pet drinks a lot at once it could cause him/her to vomit more.

- If all is well after withholding food for 24 hours, your pet is probably going to be hungry. So feed a bland diet like steamed rice and boiled white chicken for a few days.

  Note: If vomiting/diarrhea persist beyond 24 hours or you notice any blood in your pet's vomit/diarrhea, get to your veterinarian and bring a sample along!

Constipation

Constipation is when feces are not leaving your pet's body and is compacted in his/her colon.

If constipation occurs frequently, see your Veterinarian!

If this is a first time occurrence, try one of the following methods to help offer relief for your pet:

- Encourage your pet to drink more water
- Bran Cereal (no sugar type) - Add 1 tablespoon for a feline or small canine and up to 3 tablespoons for a large canine to his/her daily meal with plenty of water
- Pureed Cooked Pumpkin - Add 1 tablespoon to a feline or small canine and up to 3 tablespoons for a large canine to his/her daily meal with plenty of water

  Note: Giving felines ½-1 teaspoon of cooked pure pumpkin daily also assists in the elimination of fur balls.

- If your pet has not resumed normal bowels within 24-48 hours, see your licensed veterinarian

Bloat (Gastric Dilation & Volvulus or GDV)

Bloat is a life-threatening condition where your pet's stomach fills up with gas.

It occurs rapidly and can be fatal to your pet within 30 minutes.

It mostly occurs when or if your pet consumes large quantities of food and swallows excess air while eating. Bloating can also occur when the valve at the bottom of your pet's stomach becomes blocked. When the stomach is blocked the material produced by the digestive process cannot exit your pet's stomach.

When your pet's stomach becomes dilated/swollen or gastric dilation it presses up against other organs like the diaphragm, making it difficult for your pet to breathe. This gastric dilation makes it easier for your pet's stomach to twist, called volvulus or torsion, a quarter to a full turns onto itself.

When your pet's stomach twists or turns, all materials within your pet's stomach are prevented from entering or leaving his/her stomach. Tissue in your pet's stomach walls quickly die and your pet will have difficulty breathing because there's little room for his/her diaphragm to expand.

Fact: Bloat most often occurs in large-breed canines like Great Danes, Saint Bernards, Weimaraners and Mastiffs, but has also been seen in some small canines and felines.

The most obvious signs of Bloat are as followed:
- swollen-looking belly that appears quickly or out of nowhere
- dry heaving, Dry heaving is when your pet is trying to vomit but is only getting up saliva
- restlessness
- difficulty breathing
- collapse

Note: There are *no* recommended first-aid treatments for GDV/Bloat!
Do *not* delay getting to your licensed veterinarian!

To avoid GDV or Bloating do the following:
- Feed your pet two small meals a day. So, your pet's stomach is never over filled.
- Do *not* allow your pet to exercise for 45 minutes to an hour after eating.

When your pet runs, rolls on his/her back or moves to fast on a full stomach it can cause the stomach to swing like a pendulum and flip over.

- If your pet has been exercising, do *not* allow your pet to eat or drink until their breathing is back to normal to keep him/her from drinking to fast and taking in air.

Insect Stings and Snake Bites

Felines and canines are natural hunters and may seek out insects or snakes as prey. Just like with us/humans, canines and felines can experience an allergic reaction to insect bites or stings.
Should your pet ever experience an allergic reaction, follow the steps below:

Bee Stings

Most pets, especially canines, are bitten or stung on the face and/or in the mouth. Canines are inquisitive and will inspect an object flying or moving fast like insects.

Sometimes Canines are even stung inside the mouth because they snap at bees as they are flying in the air. It's also even possible for an animal to sit or step on a bee.

- If you can see the stinger, flick it away with your credit card or finger nail.

    Note: Do *not* attempt to pull it out with your fingers or tweezers because you may puncture the poison sac pushing the toxin to enter your pet's body.
    If you can't find it, do *not* worry! Your pet has probably already pawed it away.

- Give your pet 1 mg of *Benadryl®,* per pound of his/her body weight.

    Notes: This may make your pet sleepy preventing him/her from scratching at the sting.
    This dose can be given to your pet every 6-8 hours as needed for swelling.

- Apply a cold pack to any swelling, but remove every 5 to 10 minutes to avoid frostbite or place a washcloth between the cold pack and your pet.

If sting is in the mouth:

- Offer your pet an ice cube or ice water to help minimize any swelling.
- Flush your pet's mouth out with a teaspoon of baking soda diluted in a pint of water using an eye dropper, turkey baster or a gentle spray with a squirt bottle to help neutralize the insect's toxins and your pet's pain.

Note: Anaphylactic shock - Just like with people your pet could be highly allergic to insect toxins and may go into anaphylactic shock.

Anaphylactic shock is a severe allergic reaction that causes your pet's circulatory system to shut down.

If you notice any of the following signs or symptoms see your licensed veterinarian immediately:

1. Severe and profuse swelling

Example: Your pet's entire face is swollen, opposed to just the lips itself.

2. Difficulty breathing or increased respiratory effort
3. Very pale or blue-tinged mucous membranes known as cyanosis
4. Rapid and/or irregular pulse
5. Prolonged capillary refill time (CRT)
6. Below normal body temperature

Note: Below normal body temperature for your pet is 100.0 F

Spiders

Most spider bites can cause painful swelling and should be treated a lot like a bee or wasp stings. Several species of spiders are venomous or poisonous. If your pet's bitten by a venomous spider he/she could experience a fever, chills, have a hard time breathing and/or shock within 30 minutes to several hours from being bitten. If you suspect your pet has been bitten by a venomous or poisonous spider:

- restrain your pet's movement
- apply ice to the bite wound

Get your pet to your Veterinarian, quickly!

Fly Bites or Fly Strike

Canines with upright ears seem to be the biggest temptation for flies of all kinds. The stable fly have needle-sharp mouthparts that they use to suck blood from your pet. Fly bites don't bleed much but your pet's ear tips may get crusty form the inflammation and serum that leaks from the fly bite, after being bitten.

• Soften the scab with a warm wet washcloth. Take 2-5 minutes until the scab is softened and can be gently wiped away.

• Clean your pet's ear with an antiseptic liquid soap, like Betadine→ or Chlorhexidine.

Note: For felines, plain warm water is fine.

• Apply an antibiotic ointment on your pet's ear to help prevent from any infections.

• Ask your Veterinarian about a topical fly repellent that you can apply to your pet's ears.

Snakes

Both poisonous and non-poisonous snakes can be problematic for your pet because even snakes without venom carry bacteria in their mouth that can cause an infection.

Venom is toxic fluids created in specialized oral glands that come in two different forms:

Hemotoxic venom, disrupts the integrity of your pet's blood vessels which causes swelling as blood pushes into the tissue.

Neurotoxic venom, results in paralysis including your pet's respiratory muscles resulting in suffocation.

Here are some guidelines to help you determine what maybe a poisonous snake:
- A broad, triangular shaped head
- Vertical pupils
  - **Note:** Non-poisonous snakes have round pupils.
- Pit Vipers have heat-sensing pits on their faces between the snake's eyes and nostril which helps them locate prey.
- Two fangs which leave puncture wounds.
  - **Note:** Non-poisonous snakes leave a bite mark that is a row of teeth.

The degree of severity of any venomous snake bite depends on several factors:
- The species & size of the venomous snake
  - **Note:** Baby venomous snakes are born with fangs and venom, giving all they have in one bite.
- The size of your pet that's bitten
- The amount of venom that's injected into your pet.

Facts: Approximately 20% of snake bites are dry or no venom was injected.

50% of snake bites are severe and around 5% of them are fatal.

If your pet's struck or bitten by a snake and you're unsure of what kind of snake it was that bite your pet, it's always safer to assume it's venomous and do the following:
- Keep the snake bite wound below the level of your pet's heart to help prevent absorption to the heart.
- Keep try your pet calm
  - **Note:** The more he/she moves, the faster the venom circulates through your pet's body.
- Get your pet to the closest emergency veterinary hospital, immediately!

Note: Antivenin will be required if your pet has been bitten by a venomous snake.
- In your pet's first-aid kit should be the phone number and address for your nearest emergency veterinary hospital.

Do NOT do the following:
- Cut over the snake bite and try to suck out the snake's venom.
  Note: By cutting your pet's skin, you allow toxins to be absorbed into surrounding tissue and will make the venom spread faster!
- Try not to rub the bitten area.
- Allow your pet to move about freely.
- Place an ice pack over the snake bite wound.
  Note: By putting ice over the snake bite you will keep the toxin in one place causing extensive, irreparable tissue damage.

Facts: Antivenin is an antidote, a biological product consisting of antibodies made four common *Crotaline* or rattlesnake venoms. The antibody serum is reconstituted into an intravenous drip that is run into the patient for over 30 minutes. The antivenin is expensive, around $800 to $1000 per vile and a large canine may require 3 or 4 vials.

The vaccination is beneficial in two ways, gives you more time before death occurs or time to get to your licensed veterinarian and may even reduce the number of antivenin vials you may need if your pet is bitten by a venomous snake. For these reasons alone, the vaccination is beneficial for those who live in a rattlesnake-prone area.

Here are a few ways to prevent a snake bite:
- Stay on open paths when you're walking your pet.
- Don't let your pet sniff or dig under rocks and/or logs where snakes may hide.
- Eliminate garbage, wood piles and even ivy from your pets play areas.

Facts: Venomous snakes like Rattlesnakes, Copperheads, Coral Snakes, CottonMouths, and Water Moccasins can be found in rural areas as well as suburban areas.

Most snakes hibernate from November to March and/or in cold climates.

Low Blood Sugar (Hypoglycemia) / Fading

Low blood sugar can be caused by your pet's pancreas malfunctioning, liver disease and parasites.

The signs of Fading or low blood sugars are critical and are as followed:

- Twitching or shaking
- Head tilt
- Seizures
- Loss of consciousness
- Wooziness

~The quickest way to reverse hypoglycemia is to give your pet sugar like honey, Karo Syrup→, or pancake syrup by mouth.
Give 1 teaspoon for pets under 50 lbs. and 2 teaspoons for pets over 50 lbs.

Notes: If your pet is unconscious or can't swallow, rub the syrup on your pet's lips and gums.

If your pet is *not* alert and breathing normally within 5 to 10 minutes, see your licensed veterinarian immediately!

Muscle and Joint Injuries (Breaks, Sprains and Strains)

A broken bone requires emergency care! A broken bone is when a bone is cracked or actually separated due to a trauma event like being hit by a car. A compound fracture is a broken bone that is penetrated your pet's skin and can cause severe bleeding.

A sprain or strain occurs when your pet's ligament/leg is over-stretched. Sprain or strains often heal on their own without surgical repair but very painful for your pet. If a ligament should become torn, it will require surgical to repair your pet's ligament.

Note: If your pet shows any signs of lameness you should restrict your pet's activities to minimize the use of the injured limb.

As soon as you notice that your pet is limping do the following:
- Restrict exercise
- Apply cold compressions to help with any swelling.

Note: The compressions may be applied three to four times a day for five to ten minutes at a time.

Do *not* apply cold compressions if your pet is resistant or showing extreme pain!

- If your pet does *not* show obvious signs of improvement after 24 hours of rest and cold compressions, see your licensed veterinarian!
- If you suspect a break or can see the bone penetrating from your pet's skin or his/her limb is hanging very loosely, immobilize the limb by securing a rolled-up newspaper to a large canine's leg or a popsicle stick to a feline's or small canines limb with gauze wrap.

Note: Do *not* attempt to apply any kind of immobilization device if your pet is resistant or in extreme pain!
See your licensed veterinarian immediately!

Poisoning

Make sure your pet's environment is free of hazardous substances such as bleach or other household cleaning chemicals. Your pets depend on you to keep them safe!

Below are a few tips to keeping your pet safe:

- Examine your house & yard from your pet's point-of-view and keep all harmful items out of your pet's reach.
- Use a trash can with a lid.
- Read labels on your household cleaning chemicals for *"Pet Friendly"*.
- If you have a curious pet you may have to install childproof locks on the cabinet doors.

Canines love to chew! The spray bottles, aerosol cans and/or other chemicals/cleaners under your cabinet can be deadly to your pet if he/she punctures the container.

Note: Size does matter when it comes to poisoning of any kind! What could kill a Chihuahua or Pug may have no effect on a Saint Bernard or Great Dane.

Chocolate is most poisonous to canines and felines. Antioxidants in dark chocolates are considered well for a human's heart, but for felines and canines the darker the chocolate, the worse it is for them.

The culprit is theobromine, both a cardiac stimulant and a diuretic, which can speed up the heart while pulling fluids from your pet's body resulting in the following:

- Vomiting
- Diarrhea
- Rapid heart rate
- Seizures
- Death

The rate at which chocolate becomes toxic for your pet is as followed:

- Milk Chocolate - 1 ounce per pound of your pet's body weight
- Dark Chocolate - | ounce per pound of your pet's body weight
- Baker s (unsweetened) Chocolate - … ounce per pound of your pet's body weight
- Dry Cocoa Powder - 1/8 ounce per pound of your pet's body weight
- Cocoa Bean Mulch - If you feel your pet has ingested cocoa bean mulch,
see your licensed veterinarian!

Fun Fact: The concentration of theobromine in some cocoa bean mulch is a lot like unsweetened Baker's chocolate.

Common signs of poisoning are as followed:
- Muscle tremors or seizures
- Vomiting and/or diarrhea, with or without blood
- Drooling or foaming at the mouth, pawing at the mouth
- Redness of the skin, ears, and/or eyes
- Lethargy or anxiety
- Blisters on or around the mouth or skin
- Swelling
- Elevated or decreased heart rate
- Elevated or decreased breathing and body temperature

Make sure you have the following information in the event of a suspected poisoning:
- Phone numbers to your veterinarian and poison control nearest to you.
- ASPCA Poison Control Center Hotline Phone number: 1(888)426-4435

Fact: The ASPCA Animal Poison Control Center is your best resource for any animal poisoning-related emergency, open 24 hours a day, 7 days a week, 365 days a year.

If you think your pet may have ingested a potentially poisonous substance, call the ASPCA Animal Poison Control Center!
- Know your pet's body weight.

If you suspect that your pet has been poisoned, gather the following information:
- Determine the type of poison, how much of the poison was ingested and how long ago your pet ingested the poison.
- Check your pet's vital signs.

Reminder: Temperature, heart rate, respiration, capillary refill time, gum color
- Observe your pet's symptoms.
- Read the container label of the substance that you suspect your pet has ingested.
- Immediately call your veterinarian or poison control and do as instructed, exactly as instructed!

Note: React to the situation in a reasonable manner and try to stay calm!

Never induce vomiting unless directed to do so by your licensed veterinarian or poison control!

To Induce Vomiting:
- Give your pet 3% Hydrogen Peroxide, 1 tablespoon for every 10 - 15 lbs. of your pet's body weight, with an oral syringe or turkey baster by dribbling the liquid into his/her cheek pocket.
- Once your pet has swallowed all of the hydrogen peroxide, have him/her stand in front of you and give him/her a vigorous belly-rub, he/she should vomit within 10-15 minutes.

Note: Do *not* do this with your pet laying down!

- Collect the vomit and take it with you to your veterinarian with your pet for an exam.

Facts: Every year thousands of pets suffer or die from ingesting poisonous substances in our homes and even human food.

Many felines may love spending time pouncing in the greenery. Did you know that many species of lilies are fatal for felines? Many plants of the Lilium and Hemerocallis species are very poisoning for felines.

Commonly known is the Tiger lily, Day lily, Asiatic lily, Easter lily, or Japanese Show lily, resulting in severe acute kidney failure.

Signs of poisoning often develop within 6-12 hours of exposure.

Early signs include:
- Vomiting
- Inappetence
- Lethargy
- Dehydration

Untreated, signs worsen as acute kidney failure develops.
- Not urinating or urinating too frequently
- Not drinking or excessive thirst
- Inflammation of the pancreas may also be seen with lily poisoning

Rare signs include:
- Walking drunk
- Disorientation
- Tremors
- Seizures

Antidote and treatment for Lily poisoning: There is no antidote for lily poisoning. That being said, prompt veterinarian attention and care is necessary! The sooner you bring in your feline to the vet, the better and more efficiently your veterinarian can treat the poisoning. Decontamination is imperative in the early toxic stage, while aggressive intravenous fluid therapy, kidney function monitoring tests, and supportive care can greatly improve the prognosis. IV fluids need to be started, ideally, within 18 hours for the best prognosis for your feline.

Other ways your pet can or could be poisoned

Canines and Felines can be poisoned by toxins that are absorbed through the skin, inhaled or injected. Knowing what, where and how much your pet got into will determine what you should do to help.

- **Absorbed Poisons** are substances that get on your pet's paws pads and/or coat then absorbs through his/her skin. Poisons that get on your pet's skin or coat may also be ingested if he/she licks or grooms him/herself.

~Wash the area thoroughly with dishwashing liquid.

~See your licensed veterinarian to prevent long-term effects and to get help with discomfort or pain relief.

~For oil-based toxins like petroleum products wash with dishwashing liquid before flushing with water.

~If the poison is powdery like sink scrubs or granulated swimming pool chlorine, brush or vacuum away most of the substance before washing the area with dishwashing liquid.

~If the poison is in your pet's eye, carefully flush his/her eye with purified water or an eye wash.

- **Inhaled Poisons** includes aerosol sprays, carbon monoxide, gases, and other fumes inhaled into your pet's lungs by breathing in the poison.

~Quickly get your pet into fresh air.

~Administer Rescue Breathing, *only if needed*!

Reminder: Every other second for pet's 40 lbs. or more. But, twice as quickly for smaller pets with small, puff like breaths.

- **Injected Poisons** includes insect stings and snake bites.

Common Household Poisons:

- Alcoholic Beverages
- Antifreeze or Ethylene glycol
- Batteries
- Detergents, Fabric Softeners and Household Cleaners
- Fertilizers and Insecticides
- Snail/slug bait pellets
- Rat poisons
- People Foods   chocolate, coffee, tea, grapes & raisins, Macadamia nuts, onions, bread dough, fruit seeds & pits, gravies and high-fat foods
- Medications - over-the-counter and prescription

- Plants
- Trash

Visit www.aspca.org or www.hsus.org for a more

Prolapse

A prolapse occurs when a part of your pet's body slips or moves out of place. Injuries, illnesses and trauma may sometimes cause the breakdown of vulnerable areas of your pet's body, resulting in prolapse.

Most common protrude body parts are as followed:

- The rectum, due to straining/constipation

- The urethra, the urethra usually occurs in young male canines and generally associated with poor development of his/her urinary tract.

- Paraphimosis, paraphimosis is the inability to completely retract the penis into the sheath.

- The vagina and/or may include the uterus, due to straining and associated with birth.

- The eyes, often caused from too much pressure placed above the eye socket.

Fun Fact: Especially in canines with prominent eyes like the Pug or Pekingese.

Note: If you notice a protrusion, you should see your veterinarian!

~ Soak gauze squares with a saline solution and apply to protruding area.

Note: This will help keep your pet's organ tissues from drying out and increases the chances your veterinarian will be able to revitalize the damaged organ tissue. Plus, it will prevent your pet from chewing on the exposed organ.

~Rinse the eye with saline or sterilized water every 5 minutes to keep the eye moist until you see your licensed veterinarian.

Note: When the eyeball is displaced outside of your pet's eye socket, his/her eyelids are curled back and trapped behind your pet's eye. This is a serious condition because the eye lid cannot cover your pet's eye properly and the surface of the eye stays dry and discolored.

~For rectal prolapse, you can apply water-soluble lubricating jelly to ease discomfort or pain while you are on the way to your veterinarian's office.

Note: Your veterinarian may be able to replace the prolapsed rectum surgically.

~For the urethra, apply a water-soluble lubricating jelly to the end of the penis
~Gently move any hair that's preventing retraction.
Note and Fact: If you're uncomfortable attempting any of these procedures,
cover the urethra with a saline soaked cloth and see your veterinarian.
Paraphimosis treatment is a lot like treatment for a prolapsed urethra.
~Rinse the extruded penis with saline solution to help decrease inflammation.
~See your licensed veterinarian!
Notes: The prepuce may constrict blood flow and cause tissue death in the penis.
Apply an Elizabethan or Cone collar to prevent your pet from chewing or licking.

Punctures and Bite Wounds

Objects that pierce your pet's skin leaving small holes on the surface are considered puncture or bite wounds. With a puncture or bite wound, bacteria enters the wound and can cause an infection.
Facts: Feline bites are 10 times more likely to become infected then a canines bites.
Canine bites can create damage by tearing the skin and deep layers of muscle tissue.
Large Canines are capable of inflicting bone crushing injuries with their strong jaws.
Bite wounds on canines and felines are often disguised or hidden by their fur and can develop into an abscess if not treated right away.
Degloving injuries are when the skin is torn away with significant tissue damage and blood loss.
If blood supply is not returned to your pet's skin quickly, necrosis may occur and skin grafting may be needed.
~Stop bleeding by applying direct pressure to the wound.
~If the wound is not bleeding, rinse with saline solution or sterilized water.
Note: As the tissue heals and begins to close, the bacteria can cause an infection if you do not keep the wound clean! If an infection occurs your pet may develop a fever, be in pain, have redness, loss of appetite and/or become lethargic. Antibiotics most likely will be needed to get your pet through this!
If the wound is from an animal bite, find out if the animal, that did the biting, is current on his/her vaccinations or shots!

Facts: Felines that climb into car engines suffer Degloving injuries from fan belts.
Canines suffer Degloving injuries from animal attacks, entanglement in barbed wire fencing and being hit by cars.

Punctures to the Chest or Sucking Chest Wounds

If a chest wound exposes your pet's lungs or if there is a puncture that allows air into the chest when your pet inhales, act quickly and obtain medical assistance from the nearest licensed veterinarian. Wounds that penetrate the chest wall cavity is called *sucking chest wounds* because of the distinct sucking sound that can be heard as the pet is breathing.

~If the wound is too large for water soluble lubricating jelly, cover the wound tightly with plastic wrap to form a seal and tape it in place.

~Put a clean cloth or plastic wrap/baggie on top of the opening and hold in place with tape.

Notes: Tape 3 of the 4 sides, this will allow one side to lift up, if necessary, to allow air to escape.

On inhalation your pet's lungs push air out of the chest cavity and the plastic should lift up on the side not taped and let the air escape his/her lungs. When your pet exhales and lungs deflate in this process the sucking of the wound will pull the plastic back against the hole, preventing additional air from entering your his/her lungs.

Notes: If possible, have your pet lay on his/her injured side to keep pressure on the wound to help control bleeding and help seal the hole.

If your pet's lungs collapse, it will be very difficult for him/her to breathe.

Seizures or Convulsions

Seizures or convulsions are sudden excessive firing of nerves in the brain.

Seizures cause a series of involuntary muscle contractions and abnormal behaviors that last anywhere from seconds to minutes with a severity that can range from a glazed-over look, twitching on one side of the face, falling on his/her side, barking, using the restroom on him/herself and/or running in place. Seizures are symptoms of a neurological disorder.

Some causes of seizures are listed below but often seizures are *idiopathic.*

Note: *Idiopathic,* means the cause could *not* be determined or is unknown.

- Some poisonings
- Low blood sugar
- Brain Tumor
- Liver Disease
- Inflammation, an Infectious Disease of the Nervous System
- Epilepsy
- Head Trauma

Stages of a Seizure

- Aura - The aura stage includes restlessness, whining, shaking, salivation, affection, wandering and/or hiding.

Note: These signs may persist themself within seconds to days of a seizure.

- Ictus - Ictus is when the seizure occurs.
- Post-ictal - Post-ictal occurs immediately after the seizure. Your pet will appear confused, disoriented and may even be unresponsive.

Notes: Once a seizure starts, there's nothing you or anyone can do to stop it.
The main goal is to keep your pet from injuring him/her itself!

- Try to stay away from your pet's mouth or face, during a seizure.

Note: Your pet will *not* be in control of his/her actions and when the jaw performs involuntary muscle contractions, if you are in the way, you may get bitten.
Be Safe!

- Put blankets or pillows around your pet for cushioning to prevent further injures.
- Stay calm and make the environment around your pet calm by lower the stereo or TV and dim or turn off bright lights.
- Time the seizure, try to time all three stages of the seizure.

Note: If the seizure last longer than 5 minutes, your pet will need to see your veterinarian as soon as possible.

- During the post-ictal stage of the seizure your pet may not have control of his/her motor skills or bodily functions and might need assistance getting up or moving around.
- Do *not* leave your pet alone after a seizure!
- Make sure access to stairs or elevated/high surfaces are restricted from your pet.
- Comfort your pet with a soothing voice.

Notes: If this is a first-time seizure have your pet checked out by your veterinarian!

If multiple seizures occur within a 24-hour period, get immediate veterinary help!

Shock

Shock occurs when your pet's body doesn't get enough oxygen and is life-threatening.

When a pet is in shock their body tries to compensate for the inadequate blood and oxygen flow by increasing heart and respiratory rates, with maintaining fluids by restricting urinary output and constricting blood vessels near the skin.

Causes of shock may include heart failure, sepsis or blood infection, traumatic injury and/or blood loss. The symptoms of shock are similar to those of an pet who has over-exerted him/herself.

Symptoms may include:
- Dizziness and/or weakness
- Panting
- Rapid heart rate
- Bright red gums

Later signs include:
- Pale skin and/or gums
- Drop in body temperature
- Slow respiratory rate
- Weak or absent pulse
- Depression
- Unconsciousness

Note: If you feel your pet may be showing signs of shock, take immediate action!

- Check capillary refill time (CRT) by pressing on your pet's gums, as described earlier.

Note: If, it takes more than two seconds for color to return and/or the gums are too pale to evaluate, your pet may be in shock.

- Elevate your pet's hind quarters by placing a pillow or folded blanket/towel underneath his/her hind quarters to increase circulation.

Note: Do *not* elevate if you suspect your pet may have a broken back, your pet's head is bleeding, and/or your pet has a chest injury!

- Retain your pet's body heat by covering him/her with a sheet, towel or blanket.

Note: Make sure the sheet is underneath your pet if he/she is laying on a cold surface.

- Transport to your nearest licensed veterinarian hospital, immediately!

Closing

Developing the confidence to stay calm and effectively react is critical!
Familiarize yourself with this material and practice the techniques as often as you can. It's perfectly safe for you to practice bandaging on the your pet if he/she will allow!
If a live pet is not available you can use a stuffed animal.
Practice muzzling and restraining healthy pets until you are confident with these procedures and techniques, to be prepared for an emergency situation.
Try to make this information second nature that way when an emergency occurs, you'll know exactly what to do to help your pet!
Reminder: Do *NOT* attempt to induce vomiting, perform a choking maneuver or CPCR on a healthy pet!
Most importantly, do what you can to prevent these injuries in the first place!

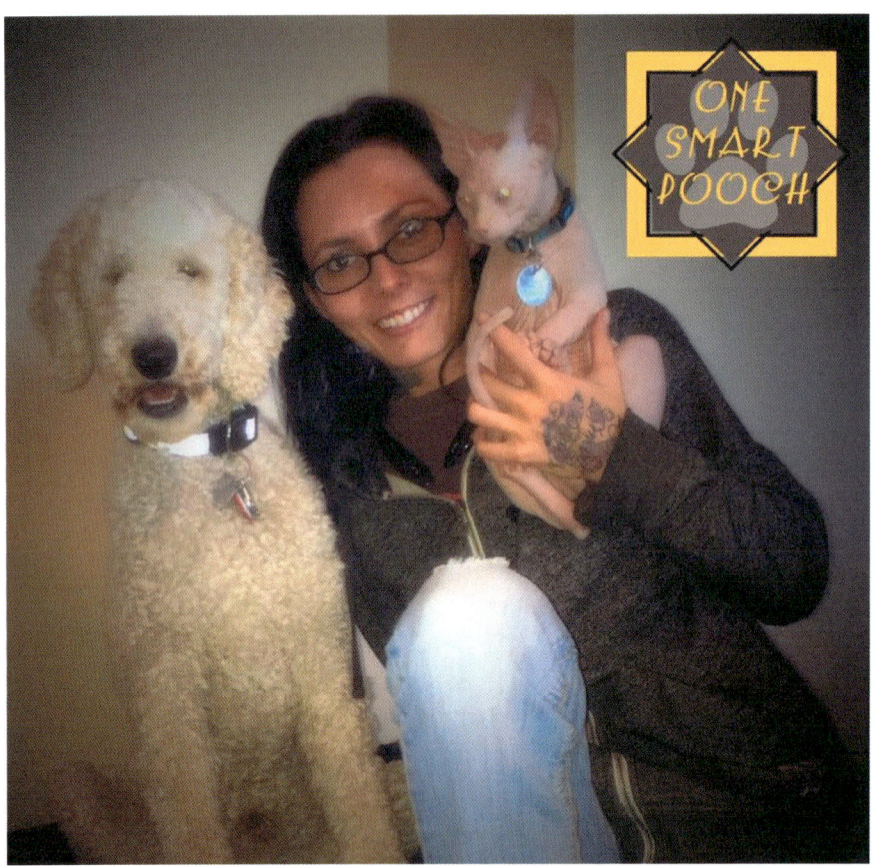

No Animals were harmed in the making of this book!
Canine Model, Teddy Ortiz, Goldendoodle, Born Feb. 2014
Feline Model, Brain Ortiz, Born July 2015

About the Arthur

I grew up in Creedmoor NC and was born at Duke Hospital, born May 1, 1987. As a child I bounced back and forth with my mom, who is no longer with us, until my beautiful grandmother took me in. I have 3 siblings, a brother and two sisters, and I'm the 2nd to oldest child. While, I lived with my grandmother I also lived with my older sister and man did we do some hair pulling, had our grandma's hands full that's for sure! Around the age of 13, when my grandmother felt I was old enough to choose where I wanted to live, I choose to go live with my mom, little sister, and cousins on the Rolling G Ranch. That is where my love and passion for animals began to grow. My mom worked 3 jobs as a single mom of 4 kids and even though the state said she couldn't have all her kids, she still had to help financially support her kids and worked a lot. So, I learnt to grow up really fast. I got my little sister ready for school, even would give up my own ride to school to ensure she went before I did, if my mom still had not returned home the next morning. Waited for my little sister to get off, helped with homework, and made dinner for her. I would like to say I played a big role in the person she's become today. I'm very proud of her and I hope my daughter, Jazmyn Marie, grows up to be just as amazing as she did! I spent a lot of time on the Ranch alone with the animals when mom was gone and the family was working on the road. I was comfort and food for the animals when the family was away. That comfort and love grow into what it is today! When I turned 17 and was ready to leave my mom's, I calling my grandmother crying after a fight me and my mom had while she was drunk asking if I could come back. Her exact words, "I told you when you left, there was no coming back!" "If you did something wrong you take your mom's ass whopping as her child because she's being my mother. But, if she is drunk out of her mind, you are almost an adult, stand up for yourself!" A few short months after we had that talk, the fights between me and mom started to get physical. So, as the "know it all" 17 year old, I was at the time, packed up my little Ford mustang jumped in with my Chihuahua and headed for the East Coast. I learnt real fast I did not know it ALL and lived in my car with my dog for 4 to 6 months before getting on my feet as a single adult on my very own.

2009, I was blessed to have my daughter, Jazmyn Marie. A year after she was born, her father and I divorced.

2010, I was lucky enough to marry my longtime friend, Julian Andrew Ortiz. He loved my daughter as his own, even calming her as his dependent through the USMC even giving her his GI Bill and retirement. Julian pushed us to do and be better! I went back to school to show my daughter an education is important. After doing high school all over with the push of my supportive husband, I decided to follow my passion for Animals and started saving up to enrolled in to Animal Behavior College to become a Certified Feline and Dog Trainer.

By 2011, I had $10,000 saved up to take ALL the classes I wanted to take that Animal Behavior College had to offer at the time and enrolled, ABC Certified Dog Trainer, ABC Certified Feline Management and Training, ABC Certified in Training Shelter Dogs, and ABC Certified in Pet Sitting and Dog Walking. As I studied, my husband's PTSD started to grow.

Mid 2012, I started working with two amazing dogs, Harley and Max, in hopes of helping my husband's PTSD. Little did I know these two amazing dogs was about to start my career! Harley was my husband's dog. I was training him just for my husband's needs! Harley was dog aggressive after a dog jumped him from behind a bush on his daily walk with my husband, Julian Andrew Ortiz. My friend, Pandora, and I spent hours on end outside correcting him every time he would growl at the dogs next door. With time and hard work, Harley's aggressive slowly went away.

In 2013, we lost my husband shortly after I was diagnosed with Cervical Cancer. After the passing of my husband I continued to work with Harley and pushed to get One Smart Pooch going with the help of my brother. Harley is now a registered service dog and I've paired him with one of my husband's brother in war. The pair is doing amazing together!

Max, was the first registered service dog that I trained. He is now retired and lives the life of a king as the only dog with the Green Family. Before the end of 2013 when Hanna came along, I was solo! Hanna is a natural at what she does! Shortly after meeting Hanna I asked her and her husband to come over and hangout for a BBQ, we hit it off right way! A few hours in, I showed Hanna what I do for a living because it was that time to walk dogs anyways. The next morning Hanna was sending me training plans for her own dogs. Had me blown away! Everything from the night before was like clockwork, a natural pro! Ever since then we have just taken off together and I don't know where One Smart Pooch would be if it was not for her!!

2014, I made the biggest decision of my life, refusing chemotherapy at a stage 3 with my cancer and moving to Colorado for a better option, MMJ. Since, moving to Colorado I'm now cancer FREE. I have continued my studies and now I'm also an AKC Evaluator and Certified in Pet First-Aid and CPR. I'm currently working on a book, One Smart Pooch's Guide through Self-Training; the book is to teach other's what I know and how to be the trainer all on your own. As I get older my body

will get weaker and when I can no longer train dogs or my soul is gone, my book and work will be left behind for my beautiful daughter to have!
-Dana L. Ortiz
Founder of One Smart Pooch
Located in Colorado Spring, CO

https://www.BecomingTheTrainer.com
https://www.facebook.com/ABC.Certified.Dog.Trainer/

Have you ever wondered what your pooch was saying?
https://www.amazon.com/Becoming-Trainer-Getting-know-pooch-ebook/dp/B071YD4CWH

Printed in Great Britain
by Amazon